Sentinel Node Biopsy in Breast Cancer

Chintamani
Editor

Sentinel Node Biopsy in Breast Cancer

Springer

Editor
Chintamani
Vardhman Mahavir Medical College
Safdarjang Hospital
New Delhi, India

ISBN 978-81-322-3992-5 ISBN 978-81-322-3994-9 (eBook)
https://doi.org/10.1007/978-81-322-3994-9

This Springer imprint is published by the registered company Springer Nature India Private Limited
The registered company address is: 7th Floor, Vijaya Building, 17 Barakhamba Road, New Delhi 110 001, India

Foreword

Sentinel Node Biopsy in Breast Cancer is a highly informative textbook edited by Professor Chintamani that addresses various issues pertaining to the sentinel node biopsy, a procedure that has had far reaching implications for the management of breast cancer. Nonetheless, following its introduction in the late twentieth century, the sentinel node biopsy procedure has also generated considerable controversy. The clinical trials that validated the sentinel node biopsy procedure, important principles of surgical technique related to the procedure, and controversies surrounding the procedure itself are highlighted in this excellent text. Each of the 11 chapters in this textbook, written by authorities in this field, provides a unique perspective on the sentinel node biopsy procedure, and the optimal surgical management of the axilla in patients with primary breast cancer.

Axillary surgery has been closely intertwined with breast cancer surgery since the late nineteenth century. Rudolf Virchow, a German pathologist, reported the results of his autopsy studies in the mid-nineteenth century, where he observed metastases to the axillary lymph nodes in patients who had eventually died of metastatic breast cancer. Based on these findings, Virchow postulated that the axillary nodes served as the nidus for the distant spread of breast cancer.

Virchow's observation intrigued the American surgeon, William Halsted. Halsted therefore proposed that the optimal surgical treatment of breast cancer should include not only extirpation of the entire breast containing the tumor, but also extirpation of the underlying pectoralis muscles and the ipsilateral axillary lymph nodes en bloc. This operation, termed the Halsted radical mastectomy, quickly became the standard treatment of breast cancer in the late nineteenth century, and the principles of that operation continue to have an enduring influence on the surgical management of breast cancer even today.

If the axillary lymph nodes did indeed serve as the nidus for the distant spread of breast cancer, then an important underlying corollary of the Virchow-Halsted hypothesis was that resection of a node-negative breast cancer should be curative. However, within a few years after widespread implementation of the Halsted radical mastectomy, it became evident that approximately 30% of patients with node-negative breast cancer went on to develop distant metastases. Thus, it was acknowledged in the twentieth century that the axillary lymph nodes were not the sole nidus for the distant spread of breast cancer, and that hematogenous spread of the tumor was also an important underlying etiology for distant metastases. Nonetheless, axillary surgery reduced the risk of local recurrences in the axilla, and many surgeons believed that it also had a potential beneficial effect in reducing mortality. Moreover, the status of the axillary nodes soon proved to be an important predictor of breast cancer outcome. Node-positive patients seemed to derive a greater absolute benefit from adjuvant systemic therapies and radiotherapy. Hence, nodal status assumed an important role for clinical decision-making for both medical oncologists and radiation oncologists during the later part of the twentieth century.

Despite its beneficial effects, axillary surgery unfortunately also clearly had adverse effects on the patient's quality of life. Bleeding, infection, nerve injury, and arm lymphedema were some of the adverse effects associated with axillary surgery. The sentinel lymph node biopsy technique was therefore introduced as a means of mitigating these risks and yet preserving the potential benefits of the axillary surgery. The sentinel node biopsy procedure has therefore had an enormous impact on improving the quality of life for breast cancer patients throughout the world.

Clearly, more work is needed to better define the role of the sentinel node biopsy in the management of breast cancer. There are some oncologists who have now called for the elimination of axillary surgery altogether (including abandonment of the sentinel node biopsy technique), arguing that tumor biomarkers and gene profiling may supplant the need for sentinel node biopsy in clinical decision making. Moreover, some have argued that, in the era of effective adjuvant systemic therapies and radiotherapy, axillary surgery provides little additional therapeutic benefit in patients with clinically node-negative tumors. Hence, there are now large clinical trials underway to assess the feasibility of abandoning the sentinel node biopsy procedure. Nonetheless, the sentinel node biopsy procedure does clearly have an important role in breast cancer management at the present time and will likely continue to play an important role in the foreseeable future. Dr. Chintamani and his colleagues have put together a textbook that delineates the role of the sentinel biopsy procedure in the years ahead, and they should be congratulated for their important contribution to improving the care of breast cancer patients throughout the world.

University of Texas Health Science Center
San Antonio, TX, USA

Ismail Jatoi

Preface

A glance at the book will be enough to take one on a journey of the evolution and the conceptual growth of approach to axilla in breast cancer. The book has richly highlighted the present evidence and newer techniques of sentinel lymph node biopsy in breast cancer which is an integral part of management of node negative axilla. The book contains the views and opinions of some of the leading lights in the field and these have been very lucidly and simply explained. The book covers a wide range of topics ranging from approach to surgical anatomy of axilla to the very recent and evolved techniques of performing sentinel lymph node biopsy in breast cancer. The reader will find the text evidence based, easy to read and understand and is meant for all surgeons and breast specialists whose heart beats for breast cancer. The algorithms, tables, figures, and charts optimally complement the text.

I would like to acknowledge the valuable contributions from all the authors in spite of their very busy professional schedules.

New Delhi, India Chintamani

Contents

About the Editor

Prof. Chintamani MS, FRCS (Ed.), FRCS (Glas.), FRCS (Irel.), FACS, FICS (SurgOncol.), FIMSA, MAMSE (American College of Surgeons), Consultant, Professor and Chief of Breast & Endocrine Unit and Former Head of the Department of Surgery, Vardhman Mahavir Medical College & Safdarjung Hospital, New Delhi. Fellow of the Royal Colleges of Surgeons of Edinburgh, England, Glasgow and Ireland; fellow, Royal Society of Medicine, UK; President & Governor, American College of Surgeons (India Chapter); and International Surgical Advisor & Examiner, the Royal College of Surgeons of Edinburgh, UK. He is also the Member of the Prestigious "Academy of Master Surgeons Educators" of the American College of Surgeons, Founding Chair "Breast Global", Editor in Chief of the "Breast Global Journal and Member of Directors" Indian Cancer Genome Atlas (ICGA).

Evolution of Sentinel Lymph Node Biopsy

1

Manu Kaushik

1.1 Introduction

"Sentinel" is described as a guard in the Oxford Dictionary, one who keeps watch or a close eye [1]. In Surgical Oncology, it can be interpreted as the lymph node that watches over the tumor. Metastasis in itself is an organised and, at the same time, progressive chaos of cells. If the sentinel node is free of disease, then the entire basin can be considered safe.

The intricate anatomy and physiology of the lymphatic system was studied since the seventeenth century with multiple investigations that have elucidated its existence and evolution. The existence of the lymphatics was first described by Bartholin [2]. It was much later in the nineteenth century that Virchow proposed the theory of lymphatic filtration. Our evolving understanding challenged the ancient Greek philosophy describing cancer as a local manifestation of a systemic problem, and such advancements led to the first radical mastectomy by Halsted [2]. The Halstedian concept of en bloc dissection in oncology lost ground with the improved understanding of oncology and lymphatics.

1.2 Understanding the Evolving History of the Sentinel Lymph Node

In the year 1951, Ernest Gould and his team from Washington Hospital centre published their groundbreaking experience regarding sentinel lymph node biopsy in tumours of the parotid [3]. During a routine parotidectomy for a benign mixed tumour, the operating team observed a node with benign appearance at the

M. Kaushik (✉)
Department of Surgery, University of Alabama at Birmingham,
Birmingham, AL, USA
e-mail: mkaushik@uabmc.edu

Chintamani (ed.), *Sentinel Node Biopsy in Breast Cancer*,
https://doi.org/10.1007/978-81-322-3994-9_1

confluence of the anterior and posterior facial vein. The node was found to be positive for tumour, and based on this histology on the frozen section, the patient underwent a radical neck dissection. For the next 6 years, 28 patients with parotid tumours had similar nodes dissected and removed before parotid surgery. These nodes were named sentinel nodes, and to their surprise, eight of these patients had malignant parotid tumours, out of which three had sentinel node biopsies that were positive and went on to have a radical neck dissection [1]. Five patients had no further surgery to the lymphatic basin because of negative sentinel nodes. The patients with malignant tumours underwent surveillance for 2–6 years, and none of the patients with untreated regional basins developed a recurrence on follow-up evaluation [1].

Twenty years later, in 1976, a South American Surgeon Ramon Cabanas presented his groundbreaking study of 100 cases of carcinoma of the penis. His work was well received at the national meeting of the Society of Surgical Oncology in New York. He located the sentinel nodes with the aid of lymphangiograms and stated that the sentinel nodes were the initial site of metastasis and might be the only lymph node involved.

If the sentinel lymph node was free of metastasis, then no further treatment was used for the regional nodes. Chiappa and his team described the testicular lymph centres using similar lymphangiograms [2]. The understanding of testicular cancer and its metastasis evolved significantly with surgical exploration of the retroperitoneum [4].

Gradually the understanding of sentinel nodes was becoming clearer and widely accepted. Donald Morton and his team studied the sentinel nodes in malignant melanoma. Initial studies were conducted on animals followed by a large case series of patients. Morton used colloidal gold for his lymphangiograms since 1977 to identify the lymphatic spread of melanomas from ambiguous sites [5]. They accurately identified the sentinel lymph node in 194 of 237 lymphatic basins in 40 specimens using patent blue V or isosulfan blue dyes, which were injected at the site of the primary melanoma [1]. Metastasis was present in 47 of the 259 sentinel node specimens, while non-sentinel nodes were the only site of metastasis in 2 of the 3079 nodes from 194 specimens with an identifiable sentinel lymph node [5]. Cabanas' work confirmed the fixed nature of the sentinel node, and this was followed by multiple studies and attempts to determine methods of its localization. Morton et al. led the way with the first description of intra-operative mapping with localization of the sentinel node utilizing the blue dye. Their team went on to publish their findings in 1992 along with the operative technique of localizing sentinel nodes in malignant melanoma.

The introduction of the dye by Morton played a crucial role in the acceptance of the concept of sentinel lymph node and the value of its biopsy. The team presented their technique at the Second International Conference in Melanoma of the World Health Organization in 1989 [6]. Tremendous efforts have been put in to identify the best technique to visualise lymphatics. Haagensen described the old anatomical studies utilizing injections of various tracer fluids in "The Lymphatics in Cancer" [7]. In the eighteenth century, Sappey et al. attempted to study the complex lymphatics of the breast using mercury injections. Guiliano published the initial paper on blue dye mapping in breast cancer in 1994 [8]. His team concluded that intra-operative mapping of the lymphatics can accurately identify the sentinel lymph node and that the axillary node was most likely to harbour metastasis in some patients with breast cancer. They predicted that this might alter the scope and role of axillary lymph node dissections. In the following years, the prognostic significance of sentinel lymph node biopsy was clearly documented by numerous studies followed by its incorporation into staging systems for melanoma by the American Joint Committee on Cancer (2001) [9]. Although its role in melanoma survival was not confirmed, further subgroup analyses provided important information regarding the prognostic relevance of the sentinel lymph node. Improvements in distant disease-free survival were also noticed in patients with intermediate thickness melanoma and nodal metastasis in patients who underwent biopsy. Such studies and findings indicated that the timing of intervention for nodal disease was a crucial factor in reducing melanoma-related distant metastasis, nodal recurrence, and mortality in cases with intermediate-thickness melanoma [10].

1.3 Sentinel Node Biopsy in Breast Cancer

Axillary lymph node status remains to be a strong prognostic factor in early-stage breast cancer, where the standard of care revolves around sentinel lymph node biopsy and its assessment of metastasis to the lymphatic basin. The understanding of the sentinel node and its influence on the approach and prognosis of breast cancer has undergone an evolution over the past century.

In the 1880s, William Halsted performed the first radical mastectomy, which became a cornerstone in the treatment of breast cancer. This radical approach was reported in 1898, and breast cancer was regarded as a localised disease. During these times, leading surgeon Rudolph Matas postulated that breast cancer is a systemic disease and might spread through blood and lymphatics. Bernard Fisher condemned such treatments and surgeons' emotions, calling the shots in breast cancer management as "almost tragic" [11]. He championed the theories to suggest breast cancer to be a systemic pathology. The twentieth century witnessed revolutionary work by physicians and surgeons in attempts to decipher breast cancer, and this has led to a complete change in the approach to Breast cancer. In recent times, there has been a constant move towards refining our approaches and techniques in managing breast cancer.

Axillary lymph node status is a critical prognostic factor in breast cancer, and sentinel node biopsy is emerging to be the prime intervention to reduce post-operative morbidity, leading to an improvement in early and long-term quality of life [12]. Sentinel node biopsy can be simply understood as the presence of orderly and predictable pattern for lymphatic drainage toward a neighbouring node basin with the functioning of the first node as a filter for tumour cells [2]. One of many initial studies on sentinel lymph node biopsy in breast cancer was published by Giuliano and team in 1994 [9]. They presented a series of 174 patients with sentinel lymph nodes localised in 114 patients. There was a positive correlation between the sentinel node and the axillary node status in 109 out of the 114 patients [1]. They postulated that primary breast carcinoma metastasises to the axilla along the pathway of nodes that cannot be identified by random axillary sampling, thus consolidating the concept that the sentinel node could be localised in breast cancer, making it predictive of the axillary lymph node status.

There is enough evidence of such sequential lymphatic dissemination with entrapment of metastasis in the first lymph node of the basin [13–15]. Kett et al. described flow to an isolated lymph node (Sorgius node) and subsequent drainage through the lymphatic vessels and nodes to the collecting ducts around the axillary vein [16]. They administered contrast medium in breast lymphatics that was visualised with the help of areolar blue dye injection.

The evolution of radiopharmaceutical methods has changed the understanding of the operating surgeon. This evolution of the understanding, along with the growing interest shown by surgeons throughout the world in the introduction of sentinel lymph node biopsy in breast cancer has led to a large number of individual series of experiences in localizing the sentinel nodes. Some series showed significance of the blue dye by itself, and some pointed towards the role and benefits of the radioisotope alone, with newer reports supporting the combination of the two techniques [17, 18].

In 2005, ASCO suggested sentinel node biopsy as the intervention of choice for evaluating status of the axillary nodes [19]. This was followed by the NCCN accepting sentinel lymph node biopsy as a standard procedure as well [20].

The introduction of the blue dye mapping by Morton et al. played a crucial role in the universal acceptance of the concept of sentinel nodes [6]. The NSANP B-32 trial demonstrated that overall survival and regional control with disease-free survival were statistically equal between the sentinel node arm with a negative node versus the sentinel node with axillary dissection arm [21]. This study also postulated that there was no significant difference in axillary recurrences between the two arms.

The ACOSOG Z0011 trial aimed at determining whether SLNB alone would be equivalent or comparable to ALND in terms of survival if there were metastases to the SLNs [22]. The study showed that early breast cancer patients with macrometastasis in ≤2 sentinel lymph nodes may avoid axillary lymph node dissection without compromising long-term survival [23]. This was further consolidated by Veronesi et al. in their 10-year single institutional data, which compared the outcomes for patients with sentinel lymph node biopsy alone versus axillary dissection [24, 25]. Morbidity was further characterised by the ALMANAC trial, which pointed out that sentinel lymph node biopsy results in significantly less morbidity in the form of lymphedema, extremity sensory loss, arm functional scores, etc. in comparison with an axillary lymph node dissection [24, 26].

The number of lymph nodes identified began to be an important factor, which led to an increase in the surgeon's efforts to identify them. An institutional study demonstrated that identifying three or more lymph nodes proved satisfactory in 86% of the patients in comparison with 57% in the ACOSOG-Z1071- and 34% in the SENTINA-controlled studies with avoidance of axillary dissection in almost half the patient population with initially positive axillary nodes [24, 27]. The SENTINA trial, however, noted a high false-negative rate when sentinel lymph node biopsy was performed after induction with neo-adjuvant chemotherapy [29]. The study noted 592 women converted from clinical node-positive to node-negative status with a sentinel node detection rate of 80% [24, 28]. On the other hand, completion of axillary lymph node dissection showed a false negative rate of SLNB to be 14.2%. When 1–2 nodes were harvested in the sentinel lymph node biopsy, the false-negative rate was 20%, indicating that harvest of fewer nodes led to a significantly higher false-negative rate. This trial was heavily critiqued because of the lack of long-term follow up, recurrence and mortality data. The ALLIANCE trial had similar results and demonstrated that the false-negative rate decreased when more than one node was harvested [29].

The evolution and acceptance of sentinel lymph node biopsy is a recent milestone in our understanding of disseminated malignancies. Its basis evolved from Halstedian surgical principles to multiple theories describing lymphatic distribution and tumour spread. The final step was the introduction of the technique of intraoperative lymphatic mapping, which has now gained validation with breast cancer patients not needing radical operations and axillary dissection with no compromise to local control and accuracy of disease staging.

References

1. Mansel RE, Khonji NI, Clarke D. History, present status and future of sentinel node biopsy in breast cancer: The Mary Beves Lecture. Acta Oncol. 2000;39(3):265–8. https://doi.org/10.1080/028418600750012998.
2. Tanis PJ, Nieweg OE, Valdés Olmos RA, Th Rutgers EJ, Kroon BB. History of sentinel node and validation of the technique. Breast Cancer Res. 2001;3(2):109–12. https://doi.org/10.1186/bcr281; Epub 2001 Jan 23.
3. Gould EA, Winship T, Philbin PH, Kerr HH. Observations on a “sentinel node” in cancer of the parotid. Cancer. 1960;13:77–8.
4. Chiappa S, Uslenghi C, Bonadonna G, Marano P, Ravasi G. Combined testicular and foot lymphangiography in testicular carcinomas. Surg Gynecol Obstet. 1966;123(1):10–4.
5. Morton DL, Wen DR, Wong JH, Economou JS, Cagle LA, Storm FK, Foshag LJ, Cochran AJ. Technical details of intraoperative lymphatic mapping for early stage melanoma. Arch Surg. 1992;127(4):392–9. https://doi.org/10.1001/archsurg.1992.01420040034005.
6. Morton DL, Wen DR, Cochran AJ. Pathophysiology of regional lymph node metastases in early melanoma studied by intraoperative mapping of the cutaneous lymphatics. Second international conference on melanoma, 1989.
7. Haagensen CD, Feind KR, Herter FP, Slanetz CA, Weinberg JA. The lymphatics in cancer. Philadelphia: WB Saunders; 1972.
8. Giuliano AE, Kirgan DM, Guenther JM, Morton DL. Lymphatic mapping and sentinel lymphadenectomy for breast cancer. Ann Surg. 1994;220(3):391–8; discussion 398–401. https://doi.org/10.1097/00000658-199409000-00015.
9. Balch CM, Buzaid AC, Soong SJ, Atkins MB, Cascinelli N, Coit DG, et al. Final version of the American Joint Committee on Cancer staging system for cutaneous melanoma. J Clin Oncol. 2001;19(16):3635–48.

10. Gonzalez A. Sentinel lymph node biopsy: past and present implications for the Management of Cutaneous Melanoma with nodal metastasis. Am J Clin Dermatol. 2018;19:24–30. https://doi.org/10.1007/s40257-018-0379-0.
11. Bland CS. The Halsted mastectomy: present illness and past history. West J Med. 1981;134(6):549–55.
12. Toesca A, Luini A, Veronesi P, Intra M, Gentilini O. Sentinel lymph node biopsy in early breast cancer: the experience of the European Institute of Oncology in special clinical scenarios. Breast Care (Basel). 2011;6(3):208–14. https://doi.org/10.1159/000329192.
13. Giuliano AE. Mapping a pathway for axillary staging: a personal perspective on the current status of sentinel lymph node dissection for breast cancer. Arch Surg. 1999;134:195–9.
14. Reintgen DS, Cruse CW, Wells KE, Berman CG, Fenske NA, Glass LF, Schroer K, Heller R, Ross MI, Lyman GH, Cox C, Rap-paport D, Seigler HF, Balch C, et al. The orderly progression of melanoma nodal metastases. Ann Surg. 1994;220:759–67.
15. Kapteijn BAE, Nieweg OE, Peterse JL, Rutgers EJT, Hart AAM, Van Dongen JA, Kroon BBR. Identification and biopsy of the sentinel lymph node in breast cancer. Eur J Surg Oncol. 1998;24:427–30.
16. Kett K, Varga G, Lukács L. Direct lymphography of the breast. Lymphology. 1970 Mar;3(1):2–12.
17. Veronesi U, Paganelli G, Galimberti V, et al. Sentinel node biopsy to avoid axillary dissection in breast cancer with clinically negative lymph nodes. Lancet. 1997;349:1864–7.
18. O'Hea BJ, Hill ADK, El-Shirbiny AM, et al. Sentinel node biopsy in breast cancer; initial experience at Memorial Sloan-Kettering Cancer Centre. J Am Coll Surg. 1998;186:423–7.
19. Lyman GH, Giuliano AE, Somerfield MR, Benson AB 3rd, Bodurka DC, Burstein HJ, Cochran AJ, Cody HS 3rd, Edge SB, Galper S, Hayman JA, Kim TY, Perkins CL, Podoloff DA, Sivasubramaniam VH, Turner RR, Wahl R, Weaver DL, Wolff AC, Winer EP, American Society of Clinical Oncology. American Society of Clinical Oncology guideline recommendations for sentinel lymph node biopsy in early-stage breast cancer. J Clin Oncol. 2005;23(30):7703–20.
20. Breast Cancer Professional Committee of Chinese Anti-cancer Association. Guidelines and specifications for the diagnosis and treatment of breast cancer of Chinese Anti-cancer Association (2019 edition). Chin J Cancer. 2019;29:609–79. https://doi.org/10.19401/j.cnki.1007-3639.2019.08.009.
21. Krag DN, Anderson SJ, Julian TB, Brown AM, Harlow SP, Costantino JP, Ashikaga T, Weaver DL, Mamounas EP, Jalovec LM, Frazier TG, Noyes RD, Robidoux A, Scarth HM, Wolmark N. Sentinel-lymph-node resection compared with conventional axillary-lymph-node dissection in clinically node-negative patients with breast cancer: overall survival findings from the NSABP B-32 randomised phase 3 trial. Lancet Oncol. 2010;11(10):927–33.
22. Giuliano AE, Hunt KK, Ballman KV, et al. Axillary dissection vs no axillary dissection in women with invasive breast cancer and sentinel node metastasis: a randomized clinical trial. JAMA. 2011;305(6):569–75.
23. Lucci A, McCall LM, Beitsch PD, Whitworth PW, Reintgen DS, Blumencranz PW, Leitch AM, Saha S, Hunt KK, Giuliano AE, American College of Surgeons Oncology Group. Surgical complications associated with sentinel lymph node dissection (SLND) plus axillary lymph node dissection compared with SLND alone in the American College of Surgeons Oncology Group Trial Z0011. J Clin Oncol. 2007;25(24):3657–63.
24. Chatterjee A, Serniak N, Czerniecki BJ. Sentinel lymph node biopsy in breast cancer: a work in progress. Cancer J. 2015;21(1):7–10. https://doi.org/10.1097/PPO.0000000000000090.
25. Veronesi U, Viale G, Paganelli G, et al. Sentinel lymph node biopsy in breast cancer: ten-year results of a randomized controlled study. Ann Surg. 2010;251(4):595–600.
26. Mansel RE, Fallowfield L, Kissin M, et al. Randomized multicenter trial of sentinel node biopsy versus standard axillary treatment in operable breast cancer: the ALMANAC trial. J Natl Cancer Inst. 2006;98(9):599–609.
27. Mamtani A, Barrio AV, King TA, et al. How often does neoadjuvant chemotherapy avoid axillary dissection in patients with histologically confirmed nodal metastases? Results of a prospective study. Ann Surg Oncol. 2016;23:3467–74.

28. Kuehn T, Bauerfeind I, Fehm T, Fleige B, Hausschild M, Helms G, Lebeau A, Liedtke C, von Minckwitz G, Nekljudova V, Schmatloch S, Schrenk P, Staebler A, Untch M. Sentinel-lymph-node biopsy in patients with breast cancer before and after neoadjuvant chemotherapy (SENTINA): a prospective, multicentre cohort study. Lancet Oncol. 2013;14(7):609–18.
29. Boughey JC, et al. Sentinel lymph node surgery after neoadjuvant chemotherapy in patients with node-positive breast cancer: the ACOSOG Z1071 (Alliance) clinical trial. JAMA. 2013;310(14):1455–61.

Surgical Anatomy of the Axilla

2

Ramanuj Mukherjee, Shouptik Basu, and Gouri Mukhopadhyay

2.1 Introduction

The muscles and fascial layers that surround the axilla are home to the lymphatics, nerves and veins that supply the upper limb. Pectoralis major, serratus anterior and latissimus dorsi are the muscles that encircle the axilla's anterior, medial and posterior walls, respectively. The only fascia seen on the lateral wall is the axillary fascia, which merges distally with the chest wall and proximally with the upper-limb fascia. This fascial layer acts as a tent to conceal the contents of the axilla because it is a latero-posterior extension of the pectoralis major muscle, which terminates in the latissimus dorsi fascia. The axilla is a typical pathway for potential metastatic involvement from breast cancer because of its complicated structure, significant lymphatic outflow from the breast and relationship to the breast. The most significant prognostic factor influencing decision-making in practically all stages of breast cancer is lymph node involvement of the axilla.

To ensure safe axillary dissection, all surgeons doing axillary surgery must be well-versed in the anatomy of axillary nerves, arteries and the arrangement of lymph nodes.

R. Mukherjee (✉)
Department of General Surgery, R.G. Kar Medical College and Hospital, Kolkata, West Bengal, India

S. Basu
Department of Surgical Oncology, All India Institute of Medical Sciences, Patna, Bihar, India

G. Mukhopadhyay
Cancer Institute Adyar (WIA), Chennai, Tamil Nadu, India

Chintamani (ed.), *Sentinel Node Biopsy in Breast Cancer*,
https://doi.org/10.1007/978-81-322-3994-9_2

2.2 Surgical Anatomy of the Axilla

The lymph nodes, loose adipose areolar tissue, axillary veins, infra-clavicular section of the brachial plexus, lateral branches of several intercostal nerves and, sporadically, the "axillary tail" of the breast are all located in the axillary fossa. Also, as stated in human anatomy, the pectoralis major muscle is encased by a fascial layer that extends laterally to create the suspensory ligament of the axilla and medially to produce the clavipectoral fascia [1, 2].

Although the standard axillary anatomy is often studied and dissected in surgery, little is known about the anatomical variants. Muscular abnormalities were found to be the most important changes in the axilla from a study of the literature for the surgical anatomy of the axillary area, with occasionally major clinical consequences. These changes, which are caused by the extra muscles in the axillary fossa, are significant for local surgical treatments such lymphadenectomy and axillary dissection for breast cancer, lymph node biopsy, reconstruction methods and axillary bypass surgeries. For instance, one of these variations, the axillary arch (axillary arch), has been noted to complicate axillary lymphadenectomy (AL) or lymph node biopsy (LNB), as well as to compress the neurovascular bundle [1–6]. Sentinel node biopsy and focused axillary dissection, which have been addressed in operative surgery textbooks [6, 7], are growing increasingly essential in surgery. The latissimus dorsi, anterior serratus and pectoralis major muscles all have unusual anatomical variations, which have been described in several anatomical research along with a few surgical studies [8].

2.3 Surgical Anatomy of Lymph Nodes of Axilla

Since the earliest stage of breast cancer spread, the gross anatomy of the axillary nodes has long piqued attention. The anatomical configuration of axillary nodes has been addressed by a number of categories. Pickren's [10] investigations, which depict the pathologic anatomy of tumour dissemination, are the most thorough. The axillary lymph nodes can be grouped as follows: the interpectoral (Rotter) nodes, lying between the pectoralis major and minor muscles along the lateral pectoral nerve; the apical or subclavicular nodes, lying medial to the pectoralis minor muscle; and the axillary vein lymph nodes, grouped along the axillary vein from the pectoralis minor muscle to the lateral limit of the axilla [11, 12]; the central nodes, which are located under the lateral border of the pectoralis major muscle and beneath the pectoralis minor muscle; and the scapular group, which consists of the nodes situated along the subscapular vessels. Other groups can be recognised, including the intramammary lymph nodes, which are present in 28% of breasts [13]; paramammary nodes, which are situated in the subcutaneous tissue over the upper, outer quadrant of the breast; and external mammary nodes, which are located over the axillary tail.

The axillary lymph nodes can be arbitrarily divided into levels during axillary dissection as an alternate means of defining metastatic spread for assessing pathologic architecture and metastatic progression [14]. Level I lymph nodes are situated lateral to the pectoralis minor muscle's lateral border, level II nodes are situated behind the pectoralis minor muscle, and level III nodes are situated medial to the pectoralis minor muscle's medial border. The only way to correctly ascertain these levels is to tag them at the moment of operation. The clinical connection of these levels with nodes that are anterior and posterior with a lateral group are typically referred to as level I nodes, whereas nodes that are central and level III as an apical group make up level II nodes.

2.4 Radiological Anatomy of a Malignant Lymph Node

It is crucial to identify a malignant lymph node because numerous benign and malignant diseases can cause the lymph nodes in the axilla to expand. Malignant lymph node identification has been made easier with the use of USG features in grey scale and color Doppler B mode. The following features are characteristic of Malignant node includes Size: Larger being more probable for malignancy:

- Shape: round
- Echogenicity: predominantly hypoechoic
- Loss of central fatty hilum/thinning of hilum
- Eccentric versus concentric thickening of the cortex
- Presence of microcalcifications
- Necrosis: cystic/coagulative
- Ill-defined capsular margins
- Heterogeneous echotexture
- Eccentric versus concentric thickening of the cortex
- Presence of microcalcifications.
- Color/power peripheral/mixed peripheral: central blood vessels, high-resistance waveform, RI > 0.8, PI >1.5 and aberrant vessels: misplaced parent vessels, subcapsular vasculature, non-perfused regions and non-tapering vessels are Doppler signs that promote malignancy. These radiologic indicators can be combined to help with pre-operative diagnosis.

2.5 Anatomy of the Axillary Vein

The extension of the basilic vein into the axilla creates the axillary vein. The brachial veins, which travel with the eponymous arteries as they climb in the axilla, and the cephalic vein, which runs through the deltopectoral groove right below the collarbone, are its principal tributaries. On the lateral edge of the first rib, the axillary vein continues as the subclavian vein.

The medial pectoral nerve, medial cord of the brachial plexus and ulnar nerve divide the axillary vein from the axillary artery. The vein is located lateral to the artery. Due to the closeness of the vein to the artery, arteriovenous malformations are frequent in this area.

2.6 Surgical Concept of Axillary Dissection with a Critical Insight of the Relevant Neuroanatomy Related to Axillary Dissection

In order to locate, stage and remove axillary lymph nodes of at least level I and II nodal groups, the axilla is cut open during an axillary dissection surgery. In order to determine if additional therapy is necessary, breast cancer is staged using an axillary dissection (axillary lymphadenectomy, axillary node sampling and axillary sentinel node biopsy) [3–5]. Individuals with operable breast cancer who are planned for any type of mastectomy are also advised to use AL. The serratus anterior muscle forms the base of the surgical field's triangle during the axillary approach, and the medial side of the humerus, where the pectoralis major and latissimus dorsi muscles converge, acts as its apex. During axillary dissection, the anatomical structures in the axillary area are anticipated to be visible [3–5, 8]. The majority of axillary dissections (lateral and posterior to the pectoralis minor muscle) comprise lymph nodes from levels I and II [3–5, 8, 9].

The surgeon will need to recognise a number of structures in order to remove these nodes without causing neurological problems, including:

- The lateral border of the pectoralis minor and major muscles
- The latissimus dorsi muscle
- The axillary vein
- The long thoracic nerve
- The thoraco-dorsal nerve
- The intercostal brachial nerves
- The lateral pectoral nerve

The long thoracic nerve (or Bell), which runs craniocaudally on the medial wall over the serratus anterior, and the neurovascular bundle to the latissimus dorsi, which runs craniocaudally on the posterior wall over the latissimus dorsi, must be identified and preserved [3–5]. In the LD-breast reconstruction approach, we base our latissimus dorsi myocutaneous flap (LD flap) on this vascular bundle, making it of particular significance [5]. Practically speaking, not all muscle abnormalities are significant for AL or axillary surgery. Only the muscle bands that cross through the axilla or alter the limits of the surgical field can have an impact on axillary dissection from a topographical standpoint (Fig. 2.1).

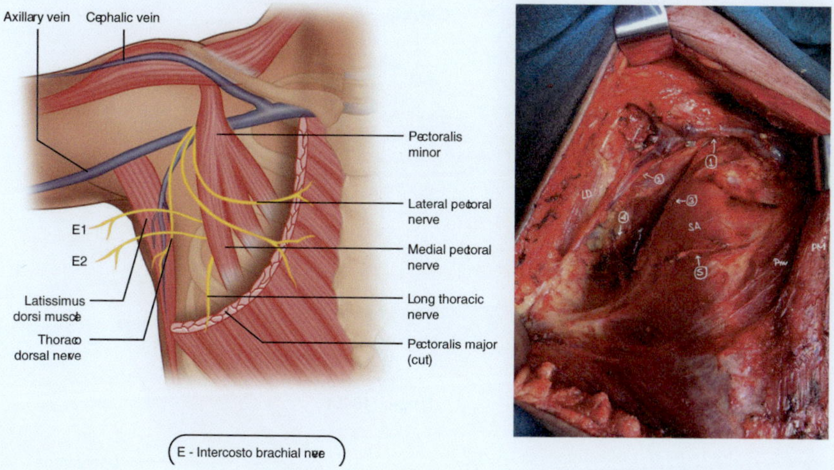

Fig. 2.1 Operative view of the right axilla during a modified radical mastectomy for carcinoma of the breast. *1*. Axillary vein. *2*. LD (latissimus dorsi) pedicle (thoraco dorsal nerve and vessels). *3*. Nerve to serratus anterior. *4*. Angular vein. *5*. Intercostobrachial nerve (cut). *PM* pectoralis major, *Pm* pectoralis minor (both retracted), *LD* latissimus dorsi muscle, *SA* serratus anterior

2.7 Anatomical Anomalies of the Axilla

Several uncommon muscles and tendonious arches, most of which originate from the pectoralis major or the latissimus dorsi and have a variety of insertions, call the axilla home. The axillary arch, pectoralis quartus and chondroepitrochlearis muscles, as well as aplasia of the lower part of the pectoralis major muscle, are three supernumerary muscles that a surgeon may encounter when performing AL, according to a review of the anatomical and surgical literature [8, 9]. These abnormal muscles are clinically significant and can occasionally result in difficulties during AL [8]. They either pass through the axilla or alter the limits of the AL surgical area. The axillopectoral or pectodorsal muscle, which was initially identified by Ramsay in 1795 and later validated by Langer in 1864, is the most prevalent. It is also referred to as Langer's axillary arch. In the literature, this supernumerary muscle is said to occur 0.25–4.8% of the time, whereas after surgery, it occurs 0.25–6.52% of the time [6, 8]. The normal axillary arch crosses the axilla and has a relatively high occurrence of 7–8% of the population, running from the posterior layer of the pectoralis major tendon to the anterior boundary of the latissimus dorsi muscle [8]. The literature describes this muscle arch as having several insertions anywhere along a line running from the pectoralis major insertion to the coracoids process. It also exhibits remarkable diversity. There have also been reports of numerous axillary arches and one axillary arch with multiple insertions (Fig. 2.2).

Although the occurrence of the pectoralis quartus muscle has been found to be high (11–16%), it is believed to be less common than the axillary arch. It is also a supernumerary muscle that runs along the pectoralis major's lateral boundary,

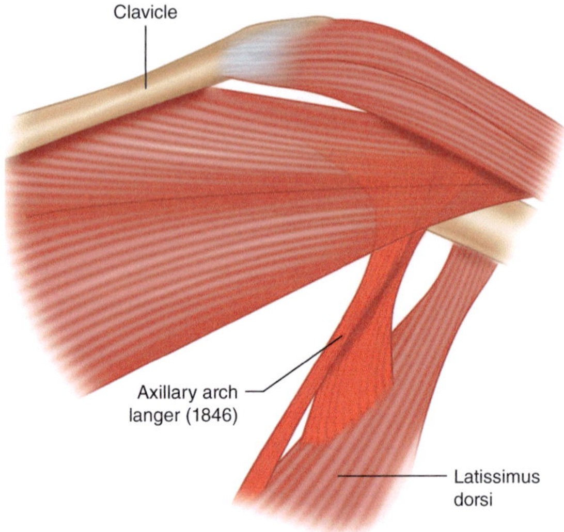

Fig. 2.2 Location of Langers Arch (Artists view)

emerging from the anatomical structures around the costochondral junction of the fifth and sixth ribs. In order to be implanted in or close to the deep layer of the pectoralis major, the pectoralis quartus must cross over the nerves and vascular bundle. The chondroepitrochlearis muscle is only sometimes mentioned in the literature, and in other places, it is said to occur 0.5% of the time. This is a very lengthy muscular band that can develop from the costal cartilages, external oblique muscle's aponeurosis, or muscle's lateral edge. It is located right below the pectoralis major muscle.

Moreover, this muscle band crosses the axilla and inserts distal to the pectoralis major tendon on the medial aspect of the humerus [8]. According to the research, pectoral muscle abnormalities affect 1:5000–1:11000 people. There have been cases of both the lower part of the sternocostal region and the abdominal component of the pectoralis major muscle being absent.

The descriptions are more frequently seen in cadaveric investigations in the literature [8]. The low incidence of surgery as described in the literature may have been attributed to a lack of awareness of the axillary arch and other aberrant muscles. This discrepancy in frequency might also be explained by the area not being fully dissected during surgery, as is the case with anatomical dissections.

2.8 Complications of Anatomical Abberations in the Axilla

Sometimes the axillary arch is palpable and might be mistaken for swollen lymph nodes or soft tissue tumours. Axillary venous thrombosis or a clinical sense of fullness within the axilla may result from this muscle arch's occasional compression of the axillary vein. The role of venous thrombosis and lymphedema associated with this has clinical importance.

Axillary arch, on the other hand, is often asymptomatic; its primary significance is the issue it might create during AL for breast cancer [7–9]. Complete axillary clearance may be compromised by the existence of axillary arch; this might prevent access to the level I axillary lymph nodes in the lower lateral group. This obviously has a big impact on local recurrence. The risk of injuring the axilla's neurovascular bundle is increased because the axillary arch may be mistaken for the lateral border of the AL, which is frequently the anterior boundary of the latissimus dorsi muscle, and utilised to guide the surgeon one level above the axillary vein [6–9]. The risk of upper-limb lymphoedema increases if the axillary arch persists after AL due to compression of the axillary vein and the lateral lymphatic trunks. Management becomes challenging in situations of local recurrence brought on by insufficient axillary clearance, and the risk for local morbidity and lymphoedema rises [6, 8, 9]. Due to the severity of these difficulties, experts have come to the conclusion that in order to perform a straightforward, secure and thorough lymphatic dissection, the axillary arch should be identified and divided to enable appropriate exposure of the axillary lymph nodes [8]. Additionally, in order to get appropriate exposure and effective hemostasis during SLNB, the identification of the axillary arch is crucial. Although axillary dissection for breast cancer is the most frequent axillary surgery, other operations in the armpit region, such bypass surgeries employing axillary arteries, may be impacted by the existence of axillary arch. Furthermore, ischemic necrosis might make LD-flap breast reconstruction more difficult if the thoracodorsal pedicle is compressed or stretched by the axillary arch [7, 8]. Failure to detect the pectoralis quartus anomaly might cause the procedure to be performed at a lower level, where the axillary vein would be placed deep under the anomalous muscle and the pectoralis major muscle [8]. The axilla is traversed by the chondroepitrochlearis muscle, which can obstruct access to the removal of axillary lymph nodes [8]. Nevertheless, the aplasia of the lower pectoralis major muscle may force the surgeon to perform the procedure at a level that increases the risk of harm to the axillary neurovascular bundle [8]. The atypical pectoralis quartus, chondroepitrochlearis and aplasia of the lower pectoralis major muscles have not been documented in any investigations, though. Thus, it is unknown what role they play in axillary surgery. Although intraoperative detection of the other three muscular variants appears to be helpful, preoperative diagnosis of these aberrant muscles is challenging [6–8]. The axillary arch, which should be detected during axillary dissection, is the only exception.

References

1. Standring S. Gray's anatomy: The anatomical basis of Clinical practice. Upper Extremity. 39th ed. Edinburgh: Elsevier. p. 962.
2. Jatoi I, Kaufmann M, Petit JY. Anatomy; chapter 2. In: Atlas of breast surgery. Berlin: Springer-Verlag; 2006. p. 7–15.
3. Jatoi I, Kaufmann M, Petit JY. Surgery for breast carcinoma; chapter 6. In: Atlas of breast surgery. Berlin: Springer-Verlag; 2006. p. 61–84.
4. Manasseh D-ME, Willey SC. Invasive carcinoma: mastectomy and staging the axilla. In: Spear SL, editor. Surgery of the breast, vol. 1. 2nd ed. Philadelphia: Lippincott Williams & Wilkins. p. 131–7.

5. Delay E. Breast reconstruction with an autologous latissimus musculocutaneous flap with and without immediate nipple reconstruction. In: Spear SL, editor. Surgery of the breast, vol. 1. 2nd ed. Philadelphia: Lippincott Williams & Wilkins. p. 631–55.
6. Uzmansel D, Kurtoglou Z, Kara A, Ozturk NC. Frequency, anatomical properties and innervation of axillary arch and its relations to the brachial plexus in human fetuses. Surg Radiol Anat. 2010;32:859–63.
7. Besana-Ciani I, Greenall MJ. Langer's axillary arch: anatomy, embryological features and surgical implications. Surgeon. 2005;3(5):325–7.
8. Natsis K, Vlasis K, Totlis T, Paraskevas G, Noussios G, Skandalakis P, Koebke J. Breast Cancer Res Treat. 2010;120:77–82.
9. Daniels IR, Quersi della Rovere G. The axillary arch of Langer- the most common muscular variation in the axilla. Breast Cancer Res Treat. 2000;59:77–80.
10. Pickren JW. Lymph node metastases in carcinoma of the female mammary gland. Bull Roswell Park Mem Inst. 1956;1:79.
11. Grossman F. Ueber die axillaren lymphdrusen. Dissert. Berlin; 1896.
12. Rotter J. Zur topographic des mammacarcinoms. Arch F Klin Chir. 1899;58:346.
13. Egan RL, McSweeney MB. Intramammary lymph nodes. Cancer. 1983;51:1838.
14. Berg JW. The significance of axillary node levels in the study of breast carcinoma. Cancer. 1955;8:776.

Defining an N0 Axilla: Pre-SNB Assessment of the Axilla

3

Susanna Polotto, Nicola Rocco, and Giuseppe Catanuto

3.1 Defining an N0 Axilla

The lymphatic system represents a part of the immune system, and it is constituted by a network of lymphatic vessels, lymph nodes (LNs), lymphatic organs and tissues. Tumoural cells are carried in the lymphatic system and trapped in the LNs, commonly metastatic sites. In the late 1800s, Sappey was the first to describe breast lymphatic drainage, demonstrating that axillary LNs collect up to 80% of the breast lymph [1].

Since breast cancer was considered a local disease until the mid-1970s, its gold standard surgical treatment was based on an extended local surgery, the Halsted radical mastectomy. For this reason, little interest was reserved to the pre-operative assessment of the axilla, as axillary lymph node dissection (ALND) was always performed, regardless of axillary involvement [2]. The pivotal point in BC research was represented by the NSABP B-04 trial, in which BC was reported for the first time to be a systemic disease with the potential to metastasise. Moreover, it demonstrated no advantage in overall survival, disease-free survival and loco-regional control for patients undergoing radical mastectomy compared with those undergoing total mastectomy (i.e. sparing axillary LNs and pectoralis major muscle) [3].

Consequently, in 1992 the sentinel lymph node biopsy (SLNB) technique was introduced and has currently replaced compulsory ALND in patients with early-stage BC and clinically negative lymph nodes (cN0). In addition, since the launch of the first trials of modern chemotherapy in the late 1960s, neo-adjuvant and

S. Polotto
Breast Surgery Unit, Guy's and St Thomas' NHS Foundation Trust, London, UK

N. Rocco
Breast Unit, Azienda Ospedaliera Universitaria Policlinico Federico II, Naples, Italy

G. Catanuto (✉)
Azienda Ospedaliera Cannizzaro, Catania, Italy

Chintamani (ed.), *Sentinel Node Biopsy in Breast Cancer*,
https://doi.org/10.1007/978-81-322-3994-9_3

adjuvant therapies have moved the focus from the most aggressive surgery to biology and patient-centred therapy [4, 5]. For all these surgical and oncological reasons, establishing the axillary status is still fundamental to plan local and systemic treatments and to predict a patient's prognosis in terms of disease-free and overall survival [6, 7].

Therefore, nowadays, every newly diagnosed BC patient undergoes a pre-operative assessment of the axilla. Moreover, recent clinical trials have proved that, in early-stage BC with no pre-operative nodal involvement (N0), de-escalating axillary surgical treatment involves no prognostic detriment. Thus, establishing the gold standard to determine cN0 is pivotal. The diagnostic methods at our disposal usually range from physical examination and ultrasound (US) scan to fine-needle aspiration cytology (FNAC) or core needle biopsy (CNB).

3.2 Physical Examination

A newly diagnosed BC patient should undergo a complete physical examination, particularly of the breast and LN regions localised in the axilla, supraclavicular and neck region. Axillary LN chain may be easily examined on clinical examination, especially in normal-weight patients.

The physical examination may be performed with the patient lying 45° on the examination couch or sitting. The first step is the external inspection of the axilla to search for any scar, bulking and skin change (i.e. unusual pigmentation, infection sign), followed by palpation of the axillary region. The physician should hold the patient's ipsilateral forearm during examination and completely support its weight, thus allowing muscular relaxation. Then, palpation is performed with the opposite physician's hand. The procedure should be performed systematically to examine the five axillary LN groups in the following order: behind the lateral edge of the pectoralis major muscle (pectoral/anterior group), the thoracic wall pointing at the axillary apex (central group), inside the latissimus dorsi lateral edge (subscapular/posterior group) and then from the inner humerus region (lateral group) to the axilla apex (infraclavicular group) [8].

It is essential to assess the presence of any palpable LN and its characteristics (i.e. site, size, shape, consistency, tenderness, mobility and overlying skin changes).

The features of typical benign LNs are size <1 cm, smooth, rounded, non-tender and mobile. Reactive enlarged LNs may be confused with malignant ones, even if they can be associated with infective symptoms and are usually smooth, rounded, tender and mobile. Furthermore, haematological diseases may occur as lymphadenopathy, needing a differential diagnosis with BC metastasis.

On the other hand, the features of LNs associated with BC metastasis are hardness, firmness, irregular shape and adherence to adjacent structures [9, 10].

The main advantages of physical examination are no healthcare costs and no pain in patients, whereas its drawbacks are its unreliability even in experienced professionals' hands.

Physical examination represents the first step in axillary staging to determine the presence of LN metastases or, if not, to assess the opportunity for the patient to undergo the SLNB procedure. However, axillary palpation is unreliable, as metastatic nodes are often not palpable, enlarged nodes may as well be cancer-free, and the technique often fails to detect deep LNs.

Several studies have demonstrated that the ranges of its specificity (between 56 and 93%) and sensitivity (between 30% and 77%) are highly variable. Majid et al. highlighted that the specificity and sensitivity values increased when T > 2 cm (80% and 81%). For this reason, many authors recommend adding US scan to physical examination of the axillary region to assess an N0 axilla, especially in early-stage BC [11–15].

3.3 Ultrasound Scan Examination

Since the development of modern US scanners in the late 1990s, the US technique has become the most common and reliable imaging modality to evaluate the status of axillary node [13, 16] pre-operatively.

US scan is usually performed with the patient lying down on the examination couch with their arm under their head. Axillary LNs are examined using a high-frequency US probe (7.5–17 MHz) [17]. US scan examines level I (inferior), II (middle), III (apical) and intramammary LNs, assessing their characteristics. The usual characteristics of normal LNs seen on US are their reniform shape, length < 10 mm, predominantly hyperechoic LN due to fat replacement, uniform hypo- or isoechoic cortex with a maximum thickness of 3 mm, central hyperechoic fatty hilum, cortical lobulations symmetrical to contralateral LNs, regular contour, painless, mobile, hypovascularised or avascularised LN and US pattern similar to surrounding structures [18–20].

Hyperplastic LNs are usually >10 mm, roundish, with decreased or normal echogenicity and heterogeneous echostructure with thick cortex; moreover, they usually disappear within a week.

As shown in Table 3.1, there is still no agreement on the gold standard US morphologic characteristics of positive LNs, even if Deurloo et al. evidenced that the best US predictor for LN metastasis for an acceptable cytology yield was the maximum cortex thickness (optimal cut-off: >2.3 mm). In contrast, Cho et al. evaluated it to be >2.5 mm [16, 37]. Other US characteristics related to metastatic LNs are peripheral hypervascularisation, hypoechoic cortex, eccentric cortical thickening, cortical thickness > 3 mm (OR = 3), fatty hilum loss (OR = 27), irregular margins (OR = 3), diameter > 10 mm, even if individually they have poor PPV [38].

The main advantages of US scan pre-operative examination are non-invasiveness, cost-effectiveness and readily available results, whereas its drawbacks include dependence on operator, equipment and patient BMI.

Many authors evaluated US scan sensibility and specificity, including their possible influencing factors. Tucker et al. stated that in patients with early-stage BC with non-palpable LNs, US could accurately assess an N0 axilla (sensitivity of 76%

Table 3.1 Sonographic criteria for metastatic axillary lymph nodes (modified by [21])

Clinical study	US criteria for metastatic axillary lymph nodes
Bruneton et al. [22]	>5 mm
Tate et al. [23]	
Vaidya et al. [24]	
Mustonen et al. [25]	Visible node
Lam et al. [26]	Round, hypoechoic node, obliteration of hilum, with or without cortical hypertrophy
Yang et al. [27]	Round, hypoechoic node, with or without eccentric cortical hypertrophy and obliteration of hilum
Verbanck et al. [28]	Round or oval node, hypoechoic, >5 mm
Bonnema et al. [29]	>5 mm, hypoechoic node, heterogeneous
Yang et al. [30]	Node with loss of hilum, eccentric cortical hypertrophy
de Kanter et al. [31]	Homogeneous or not homogeneous node
Krishnamurthy et al. [32]	Hypoechoic node with cortical thickening or eccentric lobulation
Kuenen-Boumeester et al. [33]	All visible nodes independently of pattern
Sapino et al. [34]	Round, hypoechoic node, eccentrically thickening
Damera et al. [35]	Round or oval node with cortical thickening
Deurloo et al. [16]	>5 mm or atypical cortex
Bedrosian et al. [36]	Round, oval or hypoechoic node, or with eccentric cortical lobulation

and an NPV of 89% for macrometastatic LNs). According to the authors, no patients or tumour characteristics influenced these values [39]. On the other hand, Alvarez et al. published a systematic review showing that the sensitivity and specificity of US with non-palpable nodes varied depending on which criterion was chosen for LN positivity (48.8–87.1% and 55.6–97.3% with size, 26.4–75.9% and 88.4–98.1% with morphology) [21]. US sensitivity has been reported to be also influenced by BC subtype: lobular carcinomas reportedly have a higher FNR than ductal carcinomas (13% vs 5%). Lobular cancer growth pattern infiltrates the pre-existing breast architecture, unlike ductal carcinoma, which creates a mass lesion. This pattern could also be applied to LN metastasis, explaining the increased difficulty in detecting them [40].

As a consequence of the high reliability of the US technique, several authors evidenced a significant decrease in SLNB execution after pre-operatory US assessment on non-palpable nodes ranging from 14% to 19.8% [16].

US scan plays a crucial role in guiding axillary surgical management in post-NAC settings and assessing axillary response. In fact, up to 70% of patients convert from node-positive to N0 after NAC [41, 42]. The effect of NAC on pathological LNs may lead to a partial or complete tumoural response, resulting in LN fibrosis and histiocytosis. These changes may be assessed on imaging; Hieken et al. reported a higher sensitivity for US scan when compared with MRI and PET-TC (69.8% vs 61.0% and 63.2%, respectively) [43]. Also Di Micco et al.'s study reported US scan accuracy, sensitivity and NPV higher than those of physical examination, MRI and

18-FDG PET (69.3% vs 60.0, 64.6% and 56.0%, respectively; 69.9% vs 42.7%, 41.8% and 41.4%, respectively; 73.8% vs 59.8%, 73.2% and 48.5%, respectively). They also reported these values to vary accordingly to tumour subtype (highest PPV for Luminal A and B tumours and highest NPV for HER2 and triple-negative ones), whereas Peppe et al. reported HER2-negative tumours to have the highest PPVs and HER2-positive tumours the highest NPVs [44, 45].

An advancement in US technology is represented by contrast-enhanced ultrasound (CEUS), first introduced by Omoto et al. [46]. This technique may overcome conventional grayscale US issues, improving the accuracy and feasibility of node microcirculation examination [47–50]. The CEUS technology utilises a US contrast agent (i.e. sulphur hexafluoride microbubbles) with a short enhancement time (5–67 s). With this technique, three enhancement patterns have been described: type I (homogeneous), related to histologically negative LN, and types II (heterogeneous) and III (weakly or non-enhancing), both related to histologically positive nodes, with a sensitivity of 81.8%, specificity of 86.2%, accuracy of 84.7%, PPV of 75.0% and NPV of 90.3% [48]. This novel technique may represent a promising method to assess axillary status pre-operatively. Further studies and trials are required to confirm its efficacy.

In conclusion, the axillary US scan is a highly sensitive and specific technique in the axillary LN status assessment; when suspicious LNs are found, a biopsy is recommended to confirm the diagnosis.

3.4 Fine-Needle Aspiration and Core Needle Biopsy

3.4.1 Fine-Needle Aspiration

After an initial assessment of the axillary LNs, when suspicious LNs are found, fine-needle aspiration (FNA) or CNB is routinely performed in the pre-operative setting to confirm the diagnosis.

FNAC of palpable nodes under clinical guidance has been less frequently reported and is less frequently utilised by physicians. Recent studies reported this technique to have a sensitivity between 67.4% and 86%, specificity of 100%, PPV of 100% and NPV between 62.2% and 78% [51, 52].

Ultrasound-guided FNA (UG-FNA) represents the most common method. It is usually performed using a 22–25-gauge needle and a 10–20-ml syringe; multiple samples from any suspect LN are taken, and specimens are immediately smeared on glass slices and then examined on-site under direct microscopy or via immunohistochemistry.

The average LN population is represented only by lymphoid cells (C2, corresponding to N0). On the contrary, when epithelial cell clusters are mixed or completely replaced with normal lymphoid cells, the cytological result is positive for BC metastases (C5, corresponding to N+). Other malignancies, such as melanoma metastasis and lymphomas, need a differential diagnosis with BC metastases [53].

UG-FNA represents a cost-effective and safe pre-operative approach for axillary staging. It is more frequently utilised than core biopsy as it is minimally invasive, well tolerated by patients and cost-effective and associated with on-site specimen evaluation and immediate diagnosis. Its drawbacks are low sensitivity and specificity in patients with high BMI and operator dependence, which can potentially cause inadequate sampling. Finally, UG-FNA involves a lower risk of vasculonervous axillary structure damage when compared with core biopsy and seems not to interfere with SLNB, although systematic studies are lacking [14].

UG-FNA specificity is reported to be close to 100%, and sensitivity ranges from 21% to 86%, directly related to LN involvement and primary tumour extension [54, 55]. FP may rarely occur with immune system macrophage reaction (i.e. toxoplasmosis) or benign epithelial inclusions. On the other hand, FN may also occur, especially with lobular carcinomas, isolated tumour cells or micrometastasis, as tumoural cells may dissociate in the sampling and can be missed or confused with activated lymphocytes.

Koelliker et al. reported UG-FNA to have PPV of 100% and specificity of 100%, whereas sensitivity was directly related to primary tumour size (from 56% related to T1 to 100% related to T4, mean 71–75%) [56]. Furthermore, Park et al. reported that the NPS was better for non-palpable versus palpable BC [54]. Finally, other authors reported that UG-FNA sensitivity increases according to tumour size and grade [57]. In this regard, it was highlighted that it is crucial to perform UG-FNA in patients with high-grade tumours, even in apparently N0 US axillae, due to the increased probability of associated axillary metastases [56].

The meta-analysis performed by Houssami et al. examined UG-FNAC and core biopsy accuracy in axillary staging, highlighting that the vast majority of the study analysed used only UG-FNAC (24/31). They reported a sensitivity of 79.6%, specificity of 98.3% and PPV of 97.1%. Sensitivity was reported to be directly related to the performance of UG-FNA on suspicious LNs instead of US visible ones, contrary to what other authors have affirmed [56, 58, 59].

Finally, the study by Miniero et al. examined the correlation between UG-FNA sensitivity and both tumour size and sonographic LN appearance. Whereas overall sensitivity and specificity were reported to be 59% and 100%, respectively, sensitivity appeared to be directly related to tumour size (29% in patients with primary tumours $\leq$1 cm, 50% in patients with tumours>1 to $\leq$2 cm, 69% in patients with tumours >2 to $\leq$5 cm and 100% in patients with tumours >5 cm) and US LN appearance (11% in normal LNs, 44% in indeterminate LNs and 93% in suspicious LNs). It was concluded that UG-FNA was most helpful in the pre-operative assessment of patients with large tumours (>2 cm) or abnormal LNs.

Zhong et al. have examined the association between CEUS and FNA in the axillary staging of T0-2 N0 BC patients. They reported a sensitivity of 85%, specificity of 100%, accuracy of 95.2%, PPV of 100%, NPV of 93.5%, FNR of 15% and FPR of 0%. This study confirms that most SLN-FNA-positive patients (97.1%) were macrometastatic, whereas the FN group would be included in the ACSOG Z0011 or IBCSG 23-01 criteria. Thus, CEUS-FNA may be considered a valid alternative to SLNB in early-stage BC patients [50].

3.4.2 Core Needle Biopsy

CNB is less frequently used in pre-operatory staging, as histologic evaluation is unnecessary for the diagnosis. CNB of relatively large LNs is feasible and not particularly challenging. However, CNB is not needed unless cytopathologist service is not available or in differential diagnosis with other malignancies (i.e. lymphoma or leukaemia).

CNB is performed using 14–18-gauge cutting needles and a 10–20-ml syringe. A single specimen is obtained with each needle passage, put into a formalin solution and then sent to the pathologist. The main advantage of CNB over FNA is that it allows histological examination of the specimen. The main disadvantages of this technique are the higher complication risk (i.e. haematoma, vasculonervous injuries), higher costs, need for local anaesthesia, need for patient's anticoagulation therapy to be discontinued before the procedure and patient's discomfort.

Several studies assessed that UG-FNA and CNB show comparable diagnostic accuracy. In fact, in the meta-analysis conducted by Houssami et al., even if the CNB sensitivity and specificity of histology were a little higher than those of FNA (83.4% vs 78.6% and 100% vs 98.0%), the difference was not statistically significant ($p = 0.41$) [58]. In addition, in the comparative study between the two techniques performed by Rao et al., no statistical difference in sensitivity and specificity was found. However, it is worthy to note that CNB was twice as expensive [60]. Even if other authors found a slightly higher sensitivity in CNB versus FNA (88% vs 74%), the specificity for both techniques was 100%, and CBC involved a higher complication rate (7.1% vs 1.3%) and higher costs [61].

A possible explanation of the similarity in the reliability of the two methods may rely on the sample quantity: five cores on average for CNB and 15 passes through the LN on average for FNA [60].

In conclusion, UG-FNA currently represents the gold standard technique to pre-operatively assess LN status when suspicious characteristics are found in a US scan. FNA accurately identifies N+ patients who should benefit from ALND and defines as N0 the subgroup of patients with early-stage BC who could benefit from the ACOSOG Z0011 criteria (pN0-Nmi-N1) as it is currently recognised that in these settings, ALND can be safely omitted [14, 62, 63]. On-going trials evaluate its role combined with US scan as a non-invasive alternative to SLNB.

3.5 Other Imaging Test to Pre-operatively Assess the Axillary Status

3.5.1 MRI

Breast MRI is often performed to evaluate BC extension or to assess tumour response following NAC. The axilla is usually included and can also be evaluated. Breast MRI is performed with the patient prone on a 1.5-T MRI scanner with a dedicated breast coil. A three-dimensional high-resolution T1-weighted fast gradient echo fat-suppressed sequence and a T2-weighted fat-suppressed spin-echo sequence are usually performed before administering the contrast agent. The same T1 sequence is then repeated timely after contrast agent administration. The axillary region should be fully included in the exam, and the scan should be free of motion artefacts or an inadequate signal-to-noise ratio [64, 65].

Normal LNs are smoothly contoured with a homogeneous contrast-enhancing pattern. On the other hand, metastatic LNs are associated with cortical thickening or inhomogeneity, fatty hilum loss, round shape, long-to-short axis ratio <2, comet-tail sign presence, irregular margins, perifocal oedema, heterogeneous contrast-enhancing pattern and asymmetry in size or number when compared with the contralateral side. Moreover, metastatic LNs have contrast enhancement kinetics similar to BC on MRI, with similar wash-out [66].

The main advantages of MRI versus US scan are its non-invasiveness and the axillary global view, which allows enhanced detection of abnormal LNs and comparison of both axillae. Moreover, it is a less operator-dependent technique [67]. Its main disadvantages are the need to use contrast agents, which may be harmful to patients with reduced renal function or allergic reactions. MRI is also contraindicated in patients with a pacemaker, some artificial heart valves, metallic implants or foreign bodies [68].

MRI is reported to have comparable performance to US scan for pre-operative axillary staging. Van Nijatten et al. reported an NPV between 99.1% and 99.3% for MRI versus 98.5% for US scan when evaluating cN0 patients [64].

Other authors report MRI to be slightly less accurate than a US scan [69]. As MRI is performed more often in patients undergoing NAC, studies evaluating MRI as a staging tool of the axilla are limited by mixed patient population, small sample size and inadequate visualisation of the axilla by breast MRI. In post-NAC setting, MRI is reported to have sensitivity between 62 and 65%, specificity between 80 and 100%, NPV between 44 and 78% and accuracy between 68 and 78% [70, 71]. These results may be improved by creating a protocol using enhanced breast MRI with a dedicated axillary coil in combination with T1-, T2- and T2*-weighted ultrasmall superparamagnetic iron oxide sequences [68, 72].

3.5.2 Chest CT, PET or PET-CT Scan

PET, PET/CT scan or chest TC are usually performed as staging tools in patients with advanced BC or to evaluate patient's response after NAC.

18F-FDG PET is a nuclear medicine imaging technique that produces a 3D image of functional body processes. It can detect gamma rays emitted by a radioactive tracer, which is introduced into the patient's body attached to a biologically active molecule, usually 18F-FDG. The exam is usually performed on the patient after a 6-hour fasting period. Then, a 180–240 MBq 18F-FDG is provided IV, and after a 60 ± 10 min resting time in a whole-body scanner, 3D images of tracer concentration are acquired [73].

Recently, a PET scan is commonly undertaken as PET/CT scan (i.e. a reduced-dose CT scan is taken alongside a PET scan using the same machine). As CT scans utilise two-dimensional X-rays to create a 3D image of body structures, PET/CT allows simultaneous visualisation of the body's anatomy and metabolic activity [68].

Metastatic LNs appear as soft-tissue masses, rounded and irregularly shaped with thickened cortex at CT. On the other hand, at PET an increased 18F-FDG uptake may suggest N+ LNs.

The main advantages of PET and CT techniques are their non-invasiveness and non-operator dependency. Moreover, they allow visualisation of interpectoral and level III axillary LNs. On the other hand, their main disadvantages are patients' exposure to ionising radiation, involving potential risk to the baby for pregnant patients and the possibility of allergic reaction to contrast materials containing iodine.

There are little data on PET-CT as a pre-operatory axillary assessment after NAC. Sensitivity is reported to be between 16 and 76%, specificity between 46 and 97% and accuracy between 57 and 71% [73]. Di Micco et al. reported 18-FDG PET to have higher specificity and PPV in axillary response assessment after NAC than physical examination, US scan and MRI (76.2% vs 75.3%, 68.9% and 67.2%, respectively; 70.6% vs 60.3%, 64.6% and 53.5%, respectively) [44]. Also Hieken et al. reported PET-CT to have better results in assessing axillary status after NAC vs MRI and US scan: higher specificity (84.6% vs 58.6% and 58.1%, respectively), NPV (61.1% vs 42.5% and 56.8%, respectively) and PPV (85.7% vs 75.0 and 71.0%, respectively) and accuracy (71.9% vs 60.2% and 65.1%, respectively) [43]. However, other authors reported lower percentages, assessing that neither CT nor PET/CT is sufficiently sensitive to detect metastatic axillary LNs, especially for early-stage BC [74].

Cooper et al. evaluated assessment of axillary status in early-stage BC. They reported a sensitivity of 56% and specificity of 96% for PET/CT and a sensitivity of 66% and specificity of 93% for PET alone. The sensitivity of PET for micrometastases was 11% vs 57%. They compared MRI to PET as an alternative to SLNB and concluded that MRI provided a significantly higher sensitivity and best cost-effective strategy to assess axillary status in early-stage BC [68].

3.6 Axillary Work-Up According to Guidelines

In the post-ACOSOG Z0011 era, clinical paradigms for axilla treatment have been changed, and also the role of pre-operative axillary staging has been deeply examined. On one side, some authors have argued that due to the high sensitivity of US scan and FNA, a significant percentage of patients meeting the Z0011 criteria (T1–2 BC with 1–2 positive SLNs) would be overtreated. In fact, it is reported that considering the screen-detected BC population, up to 53% of patients detected as N+ had only ≤2 positive LNs [63, 75]. On the other hand, several studies have assessed that positive axillae identified by US/FNA are usually associated with more advanced TNM status than those discovered by SLNB and associated with iN0 when considering the whole group of BC patients [76, 77]. In fact, only up to 5% of patients with N+ US/FNA met the Z0011 criteria and could have avoided ALND [39, 43, 78].

There is some discrepancy in the current guidelines about pre-operative axillary work-up for these reasons. Some centres, such as Memorial Sloan Kettering Hospital, have abandoned pre-operative US scan in patients with a negative physical examination to avoid surgical overtreatment. On the other hand, others highlight the importance of pre-operatory US scan to identify patients who would benefit from ALND [79, 80].

The AIOM guidelines recommend physical and US scan axillary LN examination of any newly diagnosed BC patient. If any suspicious axillary LN is reported, FNA or CNB is recommended to confirm the diagnosis. The same evaluation is applied before NAC to assess LN status [81].

The ASCO and Ontario Health (Cancer Care Ontario) guidelines on axillary staging in early-stage (T1–2) BC are based on the physical examination of the axilla. If negative, no further instrumental examination is needed; in reverse, a US scan is performed. A US-guided biopsy is recommended to confirm the diagnosis if abnormal LNs are found. The same evaluation is applied before NAC to assess LN status. After NAC ends, the axilla is re-staged with a physical examination. If negative, the patient undergoes SLNB; if positive, the patient undergoes ALND. Finally, for patients aged ≥70 years with a cT1N0 hormone receptor-positive and HER2-negative BC, SLNB is not required [82].

Dutch breast guidelines recommend pre-operative axillary US scan evaluation in early-stage invasive BC. If abnormal LNs are identified, ultrasound-guided CNB or FNAC are recommended to confirm the diagnosis. In particular, axillary US scan is recommended for BI-RADS 4 or 5 breast lesions and cytological punction when the LN cortex thickness is ≥2.3 mm and if the cortex is asymmetrical. Moreover, it is assessed that even if FDG-PET(-CT) does not play a decisive role in cN0 axilla staging, in patients with FDG-PET-CT N+ as unexpected finding, additional US scan with punction is indicated, and performing a direct ALND can be considered. Prior to NAC, axillary physical and US examinations are mandatory. If cN1-3, cytological confirmation is needed; if cN0, SLNB is indicated prior to NAC [83].

The NCCN guidelines recommend performing axillary LN assessment with physical examination and US scan. If palpable LNs or ≥3 sonographically suspicious LNs are found, or if NAC is forecasted with suspicious LNs, FNA/CNB is recommended to confirm the diagnosis. In patients with operable BC undergoing NAC, prior to its beginning, MRI evaluation could also be considered [74].

The NICE guidelines recommend pre-operative axillary US evaluation in case of early-stage invasive BC. If abnormal LNs are identified, USG needle sampling is recommended to confirm the diagnosis [84].

3.7 Defining an N0 Axilla in Clinical Trials

In the past, ALND represented the gold standard approach in axillary staging and was essential for BC treatment. After SLNB introduction, several trials compared the effects of SLNB alone versus completion ALND (Table 3.2). Thus, crucial importance was given to pre-operative axilla assessment as most of them enrolled cN0 patients. However, the vast majority of trials did not specify the method to assess axillary nodal status, whereas some relied on physical examination of the axilla. On the other hand, some milestone studies did not consider a pre-operative axillary status evaluation, focusing only on primary tumour dimension as inclusion criterion and surgery as LN status evaluation [90].

In the last decade, many studies examined outcomes in patients with positive SLNB (micrometastatic or up to 2 macrometastatic SLNs) who underwent SLNB alone vs completion ALND. The pre-operative axilla assessment was pivotal in this setting, as the inclusion criteria included cN0 patients. Most trials assessed axillary nodal status by physical examination, whereas others relied on US scan and FNA of suspect LNs.

The increasing use of neo-adjuvant chemotherapy (NAC) for operable BC has raised questions about optimal local therapy for axilla. Several trials explored SLNB safety in cN0 patients after NAC. Axillary status assessment prior to the initiation of NAC must be very accurate, and the inclusion criteria of trials reflect this. For example, axilla staging is performed in the GANEA 2 trial through physical examination, US scan and an FNA of suspicious nodes to assess their involvement. An LN was considered suspicious if it was >1 cm, with irregular cortical thickening and loss of fatty hilum [91]. Hunt et al. defined cN0 as the absence of palpable disease in the axilla and suspicious or abnormally appearing LNs based on imaging studies (US and CT scans) when performed [92]. Nogi et al. defined clinically node-negative axilla as the absence of palpable disease and, when assessed, the absence of abnormally appearing LNs on US scan, MRI or CT scan images. When LNs appeared suspicious on images, negativity had to be confirmed via FNA [93]. In N0 patients after NAC, SLNB is currently recommended.

Table 3.2 Clinical trials

Study and participants	Typology of patients	Typology	Intervention	Control	Pre-operative axillary evaluation	Key outcomes (primary and secondary)	Results and authors' conclusion
NSABP B-32 [85]	Clinical N0 patients with invasive BC	Randomised Phase III	Arm I (2084 pat): sentinel node resection followed by node examination then axillary dissection if positive sentinel node. No axillary dissection for negative sentinel node	Arm II (2807 pat.): sentinel node resection immediately followed by axillary dissection	Conically negative (not specified)	Primary outcome: morbidity, overall survival, disease-free survival Secondary outcomes: identify group in node-negative patients at increased risk of systemic recurrence, identify percentage of successful SLNB, measure sensitivity of SLN to determine nodal metastases	Overall survival, disease-free survival and regional control were statistically equivalent between groups. Less morbidity for the SLNB group. When the SLN is negative, SLN surgery alone with no further ALND is an appropriate, safe and effective therapy for breast cancer patients with clinically negative lymph nodes

ACOSOG z0011 [63]	Clinical T1–2 N0–1 M0, undergoing lumpectomy and whole breast irradiation	Randomised Phase III	Arm I (445 pat.): SLNB and breast radiotherapy only	Arm II (446 pat.): SLNB plus axillary lymph node dissection followed by whole-breast radiotherapy	No palpable nodes	Overall survival, morbidity, disease-free survival	In early-stage BC patients with limited pathological axillary disease (1–2 macrometastatic SLNs), there is no overall and disease-free survival advantage with completion ALND. Performing only SLNB assures less morbidity
EORTC 10981-22023 (AMAROS) [86]	Clinical T1-T2 N0 M0, with positive SLN	Randomised phase III	Arm I (744 pat.): regional nodal irradiation (RNI)	Arm II (681 pat.): ALND	No palpable nodes	Primary outcome: axillary recurrence rate Secondary outcomes: shoulder function, quality of life, axillary recurrence-free survival overall survival, disease-free survival	In early-stage BC patients with limited pathological axillary disease (at least one macrometastatic SLN), axillary recurrence was similar whether followed by ALND or radiation therapy Axillary radiotherapy results in significantly less morbidity

(continued)

Table 3.2 (continued)

Study and participants	Typology of patients	Typology	Intervention	Control	Pre-operative axillary evaluation	Key outcomes (primary and secondary)	Results and authors' conclusion
OTOASOR [87]	Clinical T1-T2 N0 M0, with positive SLN (pN1sn)	Randomised phase III	Arm I (230 pat.): regional nodal irradiation (RNI)	Arm II (244 pat.): ALND	Ultrasound of the axillary region was performed and suspected node Metastases were biopsied	Primary outcome: axillary recurrence rate Secondary outcomes: shoulder function, quality of life, axillary recurrence-free survival overall survival, disease-free survival	In early-stage BC patients with limited pathological axillary disease (at least one macrometastatic SLNs), axillary recurrence, overall survival and disease-free survival were similar whether followed by ALND or radiation therapy. Axillary radiotherapy results in significantly less morbidity Adjuvant treatment did not differ between the two groups, suggesting that pN would not change it
AATRM 048/13/2000 [88]	Clinical T < 3.5 cm, N0 M0 with micrometastatic SLN	Randomised phase III	Arm I (121 pat.): no ALND, clinical follow up	Arm II (112 pat.): ALND	Conically negative (not specified)	Disease-free survival	No difference in disease-free survival between the two groups
IBCSG 23-01 [89]	Clinical up to T2 N0 M0 with one or more micrometastatic SLNs	Randomised phase III	Arm I (469 pat.): no ALND, clinical follow up	Arm II (465 pat.): ALND	No palpable nodes	Primary outcome: disease-free survival Secondary outcome: overall survival, axillary recurrence	No difference in disease-free survival or overall survival between no ALND or ALND. Less morbidity was reported in the no ALND group

3.8 Predictive Nomograms in the Pre-operative Assessment of Axillary Status

Nomograms are graphic representations of mathematical formulas. In medicine, nomograms utilise clinical and biologic variables to create a statistical prognostic model representing each patient's probability of clinical event [94]. They are a valuable tool for the physician, evaluating the individualised risk based on disease and patient's characteristics. In particular, pre-operative nomograms assessing the risk of axillary LN metastases in BC patients may identify low-risk patients who can benefit from US scan-alone surveillance, avoiding SLNB.

US scan represents the most common radiological technique utilised to develop predictive nomograms about pre-operative axillary status in BC patients. Hu et al. evaluated patients' demographics, tumour features and BC US characteristics. Young age, high BMI, high Ki67, large tumour size, US indistinct tumour margins, presence of calcification and US aspect ratio ≥1 were associated with increased risk of N+. Based on these risk factors, they created a predictive nomogram that may enable up to 91% of low-risk patients to avoid unnecessary BLS [95].

The Skåne University Hospital (SUS) nomogram evaluated the possibility to omit SLNB in low-risk patients. Clinicopathological predictors (age, tumour size, multi-focality, lymphovascular invasion and surrogate molecular subtype) were evaluated in a non-selected cohort of patients, such as axillary pre-operative staging procedure. SUS nomogram allowed identification of the low-risk patient group with an NPV of 95%, which may lead to an SLNB reduction of up to 26% [12].

Tran et al. utilised pre-operative axillary US scan features, tumour size, grade and receptor status, creating a nomogram to predict the probability of axillary LN metastases. Utilising a probability of nodal metastases threshold <9.3%, the FNR of the nomogram was 8.7%; sensitivity, 94.0%; and specificity, 24.5% [96]. Wang et al. evaluated early-stage BC characteristics using CEUS. They concluded that high BMI, SLN US and mammography aspect ratio ≤2, CEUS enhancement type II/III, presence of lymphovascular invasion and loss of cytokeratin 5/6 expression represented independent risk factors to screen high-risk SLN metastasis patients [97].

Finally, as SLNB FNR after NAC may be high [42, 98], Liedtke et al. developed a nomogram to predict the probability of N+ axilla after NAC. They recruited patients from Arm C of the SENTINA trial and considered their tumour characteristics and post-NAC US features. ER+, multifocal tumours, presence of lymphovascular invasion and higher post-NAC US diameter were associated with a higher probability of N+ axilla. A predictive nomogram was created to predict clinically occult N+ with high accuracy [99].

Radiomics represents a quantitative approach to medical imaging, aiming at enhancing existing data through advanced mathematical analysis [100]. Zhou et al. developed a radiomics model based on grey-scale US scan images of breast tumours to predict LN metastases pre-operatively. The sensitivity and specificity of the model were reported to be 78.9% and 77.3%, respectively [101]. Also, Yu et al. created a radiomics nomogram integrating clinicopathological factors and both US scan axillary LN and BC features in early-stage BC patients to predict axillary LN status pre-operatively. The nomogram showed sensitivity and specificity of 71.9% and 81.3%, respectively. PPV and NPV were reported to be 74.7% and 79.0%, respectively [102].

3.9 Future Perspectives in Defining an N0 Axilla

Even if the current standard of care for patients with early-stage BC (cT1-2 N0) is SLNB, the possibility of utilising US scan as an independent axillary staging modality is currently examined.

A randomised trial by Cyr et al. (NCT 01821768), which compared axillary US staging with SLNB, already suggested axillary imaging as a valid non-invasive alternative to SLNB in T1-2 iN0 BC patients (NPV for US: 96.9%, no axillary recurrence in either arm of the study) [103].

Moreover, three prospective randomised trials are on-going to provide additional data on pre-operative axillary staging with US scan in early-stage N0 BC. Their unifying purpose is to compare observation with SLNB in patients with early-stage BC undergoing BCS and adjuvant radiation therapy.

The SOUND trial enrolled iT1cN0M0 patients whose axilla was evaluated with US scan±FNAC. Patients were randomised to either no axillary surgical staging or SLNB±ALND. Trial endpoints were the distant disease-free survival, distant recurrences, axillary recurrences, DFS, OS and quality of life [104].

INSEMA is a double-randomisation trial that enrolled iT1/iT2cN0M0 patients whose axillae were evaluated with physical examination and US scan±FNAC/CNB. The patients were randomised to either no axillary surgical staging or SLNB. In this second group, if the final pathology was for up to 3 macrometastatic LNs, they were furtherly randomized to SLNB alone Vs completion ALND. The trial endpoint was invasive disease-free survival (IDFS) [105].

Finally, BOOG 2013-08 enrolled iT1/iT2cN0M0 patients, including those who had undergone NAC. Axillary status was evaluated with physical examination and US scan±FNAC/CNB. The patients were randomised to either no axillary surgical staging or SLNB±ALND. The trial endpoint was the regional recurrence rate [106].

References

1. Reynolds HM, Walker CG, Dunbar PR, et al. Functional anatomy of the lymphatics draining the skin: a detailed statistical analysis. J Anat. 2010;216(3):344–55. https://doi.org/10.1111/j.1469-7580.2009.01183.
2. Halsted WS. I. The results of radical operations for the cure of carcinoma of the breast. Ann Surg. 1907;46(1):1–19.
3. Fisher B, Jeong JH, Anderson S, et al. Twenty-five-year follow-up of a randomized trial comparing radical mastectomy, total mastectomy, and total mastectomy followed by irradiation. N Engl J Med. 2002;347(8):567–75. https://doi.org/10.1056/NEJMoa020128.

4. Bonadonna G, Brusamolino E, Valagussa P, et al. Combined chemotherapy as adjuvant treatment in operable breast cancer. N Engl J Med. 1976;294:405–10.
5. Bonadonna G, Veronesi U, Brambilla C, et al. Primary chemotherapy to avoid mastectomy in tumors with diameters of three centimeters or more. J Natl Cancer Inst. 1990;82:1539–45.
6. (TNM) National Comprehensive Cancer Network. Invasive breast cancer (Version 6.2020). https://www.nccn.org/professionals/physician_gls/pdf/breast.pdf. Accessed 12 Nov 2020.
7. Burstein HJ, Curigliano G, Loibl S, et al. Estimating the benefits of therapy for early-stage breast cancer: the St. Gallen international consensus guidelines for the primary therapy of early breast cancer 2019. Ann Oncol. 2019;30(10):1541–57. https://doi.org/10.1093/annonc/mdz235.
8. Bates' guide to physical examination and history taking. Philadelphia: Wolters Kluwer Health/Lippincott Williams & Wilkins; 2009.
9. Bromberg M. Assessment of lymphadenopathy. In: BMJ best practice; 2017. https://bestpractice.bmj.com/topics/en-gb/838.
10. Rosenberg S. Lymph node exam findings stanford.edu. https://stanfordmedicine25.stanford.edu/the25/lymph.html.
11. Lanng C, Hoffmann J, Galatius H, et al. Assessment of clinical palpation of the axilla as a criterion for performing the sentinel node procedure in breast cancer. Eur J Surg Oncol. 2007;33(3):281–4. https://doi.org/10.1016/j.ejso.2006.09.032; Epub 2006 Nov 3.
12. Majid S, Bendahl PO, Huss L, et al. Validation of the Skåne University Hospital nomogram for the preoperative prediction of a disease-free axilla in patients with breast cancer. BJS Open. 2021;5(3):zrab027. https://doi.org/10.1093/bjsopen/zrab027.
13. de Freitas R, Costa MV, Schneider SV, et al. Accuracy of ultrasound and clinical examination in the diagnosis of axillary lymph node metastases in breast cancer. Eur J Surg Oncol. 1991;17:240–4.
14. Sauer T, Suciu V. The role of preoperative axillary lymph node fine needle aspiration in locoregional staging of breast cancer. Ann Pathol. 2012;32(6):e24–8, 410–4. English, French. https://doi.org/10.1016/j.annpat.2012.09.229.
15. Specht MC, Fey JV, Borgen PI, et al. Is the clinically positive axilla in breast cancer really a contraindication to sentinel lymph node biopsy? J Am Coll Surg. 2005;200:10–4.
16. Deurloo EE, Tanis PJ, Gilhuijs KG, et al. Reduction in the number of sentinel lymph node procedures by preoperative ultrasonography of the axilla in breast cancer. Eur J Cancer. 2003;39(8):1068–73. https://doi.org/10.1016/s0959-8049(02)00748-7.
17. Dialani V, James DF, Slanetz PJ. A practical approach to imaging the axilla. Insights Imaging. 2015;6(2):217–29. https://doi.org/10.1007/s13244-014-0367-824.
18. Net JM, Mirpuri TM, Plaza MJ, et al. Resident and fellow education feature: US evaluation of axillary lymph nodes. Radiographics. 2014;34(7):1817–8. https://doi.org/10.1148/rg.347140081.
19. Britton PD, Goud A, Godward S, et al. Use of ultrasound- guided axillary node core biopsy in staging of early breast cancer. Eur Radiol. 2009;19:561–9.
20. Sencha AN, et al. Breast ultrasound. Berlin: Springer-Verlag; 2013. https://doi.org/10.1007/978-3-642-36502-7_10.
21. Alvarez S, Anorbe E, Alcorta P, et al. Role of sonography in the diagnosis of axillary lymph node metastases in breast cancer: a systematic review. AJR Am J Roentgenol. 2006;186:1342–8.
22. Bruneton JN, Caramella E, Héry M, et al. Axillary lymph node metastases in breast cancer: preoperative detection with US. Radiology. 1986;158:325–6.
23. Tate JJ, Lewis V, Archer T, et al. Ultrasound detection of axillary lymph node metastases in breast cancer. Eur J Surg Oncol. 1989;15:139–41.
24. Vaidya JS, Vyas JJ, Thakur MH, et al. Role of ultrasonography to detect axillary node involvement in operable breast cancer. Eur J Surg Oncol. 1996;22:140–3.
25. Mustonen P, Farin P, Kosunen O. Ultrasonographic detection of metastatic axillary lymph nodes in breast cancer. Ann Chir Gynaecol. 1990;79:15–8.

26. Lam WW, Yang WT, Chan YL, et al. Detection of axillary lymph node metastases in breast carcinoma by technetium-99m sestamibi breast scintigraphy, ultrasound and conventional mammography. Eur J Nucl Med. 1996;23:498–503.
27. Yang WT, Ahuja A, Tang A, et al. High resolution sonographic detection of axillary lymph node metastases in breast cancer. J Ultrasound Med. 1996;16:241–6; erratum in: J Ultrasound Med 1996; 15:644.
28. Verbanck J, Vandewiele I, De Winter H, et al. Value of axillary ultrasonography and sonographically guided needle biopsy of axillary nodes: a prospective study in 144 consecutive patients. J Clin Ultrasound. 1997;25:53–6.
29. Bonnema J, van Geel AN, van Ooijen B, et al. Ultrasound-guided aspiration biopsy for detection of nonpalpable axillary node metastases in breast cancer patients: new diagnostic method. World J Surg. 1997;21:270–4.
30. Yang WT, Metreweli C. Colour Doppler flow in normal axillary lymph nodes. Br J Radiol. 1998;71:381–3.
31. de Kanter AY, van Eijck CH, van Geel AN, et al. Multicentre study of ultrasonographically guided axillary node biopsy in patients with breast cancer. Br J Surg. 1999;86:1459–62.
32. Krishnamurthy S, Sneige N, Bedi DG, et al. Role of ultrasound-guided fine-needle aspiration of indeterminate and suspicious axillary lymph nodes in the initial staging of breast carcinoma. Cancer. 2002;95:982–8.
33. Kuenen-Boumeester V, Menke-Pluymers M, de Kanter AY, et al. Ultrasound-guided fine needle aspiration cytology of axillary lymph nodes in breast cancer patients: a preoperative staging procedure. Eur J Cancer. 2003;39:170–4.
34. Sapino A, Cassoni P, Zanon E, et al. Ultrasonographically-guided fine-needle aspiration of axillary lymph nodes: role in breast cancer management. Br J Cancer. 2003;88:702–6.
35. Damera A, Evans AJ, Cornford EJ, et al. Diagnosis of axillary nodal metastases by ultrasound-guided core biopsy in primary operable breast cancer. Br J Cancer. 2003;89:1310–3.
36. Bedrosian I, Bedi D, Kuerer HM, et al. Impact of clinicopathological factors on sensitivity of axillary ultrasonography in the detection of axillary nodal metastases in patients with breast cancer. Ann Surg Oncol. 2003;10:1025–30.
37. Cho N, Moon WK, Han W, et al. Preoperative sonographic classification of axillary lymph nodes in patients with breast cancer: node-to-node correlation with surgical histology and sentinel node biopsy results. AJR Am J Roentgenol. 2009;193:1731–7.
38. Chen MY, Gillanders WE. Staging of the axilla in breast cancer and the evolving role of axillary ultrasound. Breast Cancer (Dove Med Press). 2021;13:311–23. https://doi.org/10.2147/BCTT.S273039.
39. Tucker NS, Cyr AE, Ademuyiwa FO, et al. Axillary ultrasound accurately excludes clinically significant lymph node disease in patients with early stage breast cancer. Ann Surg. 2015;264:1098.
40. Johnson S, Brown S, Porter G, et al. Staging primary breast cancer. Are there tumour pathological features that correlate with a false-negative axillary ultrasound? Clin Radiol. 2011;66:497–9.
41. Boughey JC, Ballman KV, Hunt KK, et al. Axillary ultrasound after neoadjuvant chemotherapy and its impact on sentinel lymph node surgery: results from the American College of Surgeons Oncology Group Z1071 Trial (Alliance). J Clin Oncol. 2015;33(30):3386–93. https://doi.org/10.1200/JCO.2014.57.840146.
42. Boughey JC, Suman VJ, Mittendorf EA, et al. The role of sentinel lymph node surgery in patients presenting with node positive breast cancer (T0–T4, N1–2) who receive neoadjuvant chemotherapy—results from the ACOSOG Z1071 trial (abstract). Cancer Res. 2012;72:S2–1.
43. Hieken TJ, Boughey JC, Jones KN, et al. Imaging response and residual metastatic axillary lymph node disease after neoadjuvant chemotherapy for primary breast cancer. Ann Surg Oncol. 2013;20(10):3199–204. https://doi.org/10.1245/s10434-013-3118-z.
44. Di Micco R, Zuber V, Fiacco E, et al. Sentinel node biopsy after primary systemic therapy in node positive breast cancer patients: time trend, imaging staging power and nodal down-

staging according to molecular subtype. Eur J Surg Oncol. 2019;45(6):969–75. https://doi.org/10.1016/j.ejso.2019.01.21948.

45. Peppe A, Wilson R, Pope R, et al. The use of ultrasound in the clinical re-staging of the axilla after neoadjuvant chemotherapy (NACT). Breast. 2017;35:104e8.
46. Omoto K, Hozumi Y, Omoto Y, et al. Sentinel node detection in breast cancer using contrast-enhanced sonography with 25% albumin —initial clinical experience. J Clin Ultrasound. 2006;34(7):317–26. https://doi.org/10.1002/jcu.20241.
47. Xu HX. Contrast-enhanced ultrasound: the evolving applications. World J Radiol. 2009;1:15–24.
48. Xie F, Zhang D, Cheng L, et al. Intradermal microbubbles and contrast-enhanced ultrasound (CEUS) is a feasible approach for sentinel lymph node identification in early-stage breast cancer. World J Surg Oncol. 2015;13:319. https://doi.org/10.1186/s12957-015-0736-x.
49. Dellaportas D, Koureas A, Contis J, et al. Contrast-enhanced color Doppler ultrasonography for preoperative evaluation of sentinel lymph node in breast cancer patients. Breast Care (Basel). 2015;10(5):331–5. https://doi.org/10.1159/000436958; Epub 2015 Jul 10.
50. Zhong J, Sun DS, Wei W, et al. Contrast-enhanced ultrasound-guided fine-needle aspiration for sentinel lymph node biopsy in early-stage breast cancer. Ultrasound Med Biol. 2018;44(7):1371–8. https://doi.org/10.1016/j.ultrasmedbio.2018.03.005; Epub 2018 Apr 6.
51. Marti JL, Ayo D, Levine P, et al. Nonimage-guided fine needle aspiration biopsy of palpable axillary lymph nodes in breast cancer patients. Breast J. 2012;18:3–7.
52. Alkuwari E, Auger M. Accuracy of fine-needle aspiration cytology of axillary lymph nodes in breast cancer patients: a study of 115 cases with cytologic-histologic correlation. Cancer. 2008;114:89–93.
53. O'Malley FP, Pinder SE, Mulligan AM. Breast pathology E-Book: a volume in the series: Foundations in diagnostic pathology. Edinburgh: Churchill Livingstone; 2011.
54. Park SH, Kim MJ, Park BW, et al. Impact of preoperative ultrasonography and fine-needle aspiration of axillary lymph nodes on surgical management of primary breast cancer. Ann Surg Oncol. 2011;18:738–44.
55. van Rijk MC, Deurloo EE, Nieweg OE, et al. Ultrasonography and fine-needle aspiration cytology can spare breast cancer patients unnecessary sentinel lymph node biopsy. Ann Surg Oncol. 2006;13:31–5.
56. Koelliker SL, Chung MA, Mainiero MB, et al. Axillary lymph nodes: US-guided fine-needle aspiration for initial staging of breast cancer-correlation with primary tumor size. Radiology. 2008;246:81–9.
57. Baruah BP, Goyal A, Young P, et al. Axillary node staging by ultrasonography and fine-needle aspiration cytology in patients with breast cancer. Br J Surg. 2010;97:680–3.
58. Houssami N, Ciatto S, Turner RM, et al. Preoperative US-guided needle biopsy of axillary nodes in invasive breast cancer. Meta-analysis of its accuracy and utility in staging the axilla. Ann Surg. 2011;254:243–51.
59. Jain A, Haisfield-Wolfe ME, Lange J, et al. The role of ultrasound-guided fine needle aspiration of axillary nodes in the staging of breast cancer. Ann Surg Oncol. 2008;15:462–71.
60. Rao R, Lilley L, Andrews V, et al. Axillary staging by percutaneous biopsy: sensitivity of fine-needle aspiration versus core needle biopsy. Ann Surg Oncol. 2009;16:1170–5.
61. Balasubramanian I, Fleming CA, Corrigan MA, et al. Meta-analysis of the diagnostic accuracy of ultrasound-guided fine-needle aspiration and core needle biopsy in diagnosing axillary lymph node metastasis. Br J Surg. 2018;105(10):1244–53. https://doi.org/10.1002/bjs.10920; Epub 2018 Jul 4.
62. Cangiarella J, Simsir A, Tabbara SO. Breast cytohistology. Cambridge: Cambridge University Press; 2013.
63. Giuliano AE, Ballman KV, McCall L, et al. Effect of axillary dissection vs no axillary dissection on 10-year overall survival among women with invasive breast cancer and sentinel node metastasis: the ACOSOG Z0011 (Alliance) randomized clinical trial. JAMA. 2017;318(10):918–26. https://doi.org/10.1001/jama.2017.11470.

64. van Nijnatten TJA, Ploumen EH, Schipper RJ, et al. Routine use of standard breast MRI compared to axillary ultrasound for differentiating between no, limited and advanced axillary nodal disease in newly diagnosed breast cancer patients. Eur J Radiol. 2016;85(12):2288–94.
65. Arslan G, et al. Diagnostic accuracy of metastatic axillary lymph nodes in breast MRI. Springerplus. 2016;5(1):735. https://doi.org/10.1186/s40064-016-2419-7.
66. Kvistad KA, Rydland J, Smethurst HB, et al. Axillary lymph node metastases in breast cancer: preoperative detection with dynamic contrast-enhanced MRI. Eur Radiol. 2000;10(9):1464–71. https://doi.org/10.1007/s003300000370.
67. Chang JM, Leung JWT, Moy L, et al. Axillary nodal evaluation in breast cancer: state of the art. Radiology. 2020;295(3):500–15. https://doi.org/10.1148/radiol.2020192534; Epub 2020 Apr 21.
68. Cooper KL, Meng Y, Harnan S, et al. Positron emission tomography (PET) and magnetic resonance imaging (MRI) for the assessment of axillary lymph node metastases in early breast cancer: systematic review and economic evaluation. Health Technol Assess. 2011;15(4):iii–v, 1–134. https://doi.org/10.3310/hta15040.
69. Ramirez SI, Scholle M, Buckmaster J, et al. Assessment of the accuracy of ultrasound compared to magnetic resonance imaging in the ability to detect metastatic breast cancer to the axilla (abstract). Surg Tech Dev. 2012;2. https://doi.org/10.4081/std.2012.e4.
70. Javid S, Segara D, Lotfi P, et al. Can breast MRI predict axillary lymph node metastasis in women undergoing neoadjuvant chemotherapy? Ann Surg Oncol. 2010;17:1841–6.
71. Williams A, Litton KJ, Borley A, et al. Imaging the breast following neoadjuvant chemotherapy: does improvement of imaging findings in the axilla predict pathological response in the breast? Breast Cancer Res. 2012;14(Suppl 1):P30.
72. Kuijs VJL, Moossdorff M, Schipper RJ, et al. The role of MRI in axillary lymph node imaging in breast cancer patients: a systematic review. Insights Imaging. 2015;6:203–15. https://doi.org/10.1007/s13244-015-0404-2.
73. Koolen BB, Valdés Olmos RA, Wesseling J, et al. Early assessment of axillary response with ^{18}F-FDG PET/CT during neoadjuvant chemotherapy in stage II-III breast cancer: implications for surgical management of the axilla. Ann Surg Oncol. 2013;20(7):2227–35. https://doi.org/10.1245/s10434-013-2902-0; Epub 2013 Mar 1.
74. NCCN Guidelines Version 2.2022 Breast Cancer. www.nccn.org.
75. Wallis MG, Kilburn-Toppin F, Taylor-Phillips S. Does preoperative axillary staging lead to overtreatment of women with screen-detected breast cancer? Clin Radiol. 2018;73(5):467–72.
76. Verheuvel NC, van den Hoven I, Ooms HW, et al. The role of ultrasound-guided lymph node biopsy in axillary staging of invasive breast cancer in the post-ACOSOG Z0011 trial era. Ann Surg Oncol. 2015;22(2):409–15. https://doi.org/10.1245/s10434-014-4071-1.
77. Caudle AS, Kuerer HM, Le-petross HT, et al. Predicting the extent of nodal disease in early-stage breast cancer. Ann Surg Oncol. 2014;21(11):3440–7. https://doi.org/10.1245/s10434-014-3813-4.
78. Joh JE, Han G, Kiluk JV, et al. Indications for axillary ultrasound use in breast cancer patients. Clin Breast Cancer. 2012;12(6):433–7. https://doi.org/10.1016/j.clbc.2012.09.009.
79. Boland MR, Prichard RS, Daskalova I, et al. Axillary nodal burden in primary breast cancer patients with positive preoperative ultrasound guided fine needle aspiration cytology: management in the era of ACOSOG Z0011. Eur J Surg Oncol. 2015;41(4):559–65.
80. Reyna C, Kiluk JV, Frelick A, et al. Impact of axillary ultrasound (AUS) on axillary dissection in breast conserving surgery (BCS). J Surg Oncol. 2015;111:813e8.
81. AIOM. Associazione Italiana di Oncologia Medica. Linee guida NEOPLASIE DELLA MAMMELLA. Edizione 2020. https://www.aiom.it/.
82. Brackstone M, Baldassarre FG, Perera FE, et al. Management of the Axilla in early-stage breast cancer: Ontario Health (Cancer Care Ontario) and ASCO guideline. J Clin Oncol. 2021;39(27):3056–82. https://doi.org/10.1200/JCO.21.00934; Epub 2021 Jul 19.
83. Breast cancer. Dutch Guideline, version 2.0. https://www.oncoline.nl/uploaded/docs/mammacarcinoom/Dutch%20Breast%20Cancer%20Guideline%202012.pdf.

84. Early and locally advanced breast cancer: diagnosis and management. NICE guideline. Published: 18 July 2018. www.nice.org.uk/guidance/ng101.
85. Krag DN, Anderson SJ, Julian TB, et al. Sentinel-lymph-node resection compared with conventional axillary-lymph-node dissection in clinically node-negative patients with breast cancer: overall survival findings from the NSABP B-32 randomised phase 3 trial. Lancet Oncol. 2010;11(10):927–33. https://doi.org/10.1016/S1470-2045(10)70207-2.
86. Donker M, van Tienhoven G, Straver ME, et al. Radiotherapy or surgery of the axilla after a positive sentinel node in breast cancer (EORTC 10981–22023 AMAROS): a randomised, multicentre, open-label, phase 3 non-inferiority trial. Lancet Oncol. 2014;15(12):1303–10. https://doi.org/10.1016/S1470-2045(14)70460-7; Epub 2014 Oct 15.
87. Sávolt Á, Péley G, Polgár C, et al. Eight-year follow up result of the OTOASOR trial: the optimal treatment of the axilla - surgery or radiotherapy after positive sentinel lymph node biopsy in early-stage breast cancer: a randomized, single centre, phase III, non-inferiority trial. Eur J Surg Oncol. 2017;43(4):672–9. https://doi.org/10.1016/j.ejso.2016.12.011; Epub 2017 Jan 16.
88. Solá M, Alberro JA, Fraile M, et al. Complete axillary lymph node dissection versus clinical follow-up in breast cancer patients with sentinel node micrometastasis: final results from the multicenter clinical trial AATRM 048/13/2000. Ann Surg Oncol. 2013;20(1):120–7. https://doi.org/10.1245/s10434-012-2569-y; Epub 2012 Sep 7.
89. Galimberti V, Cole BF, Viale G, et al. International Breast Cancer Study Group Trial 23-01. Axillary dissection versus no axillary dissection in patients with breast cancer and sentinel-node micrometastases (IBCSG 23-01): 10-year follow-up of a randomised, controlled phase 3 trial. Lancet Oncol. 2018;19(10):1385–93. https://doi.org/10.1016/S1470-2045(18)30380-2; Epub 2018 Sep 5.
90. Veronesi U, Viale G, Paganelli G, et al. Sentinel lymph node biopsy in breast cancer: ten-year results of a randomized controlled study. Ann Surg. 2010;251:595–600.
91. Classe JM, Loaec C, Gimbergues P, et al. Sentinel lymph node biopsy without axillary lymphadenectomy after neoadjuvant chemotherapy is accurate and safe for selected patients: the GANEA 2 study. Breast Cancer Res Treat. 2019;173(2):343–52. https://doi.org/10.1007/s10549-018-5004-7; Epub 2018 Oct 20.
92. Hunt KK, Ballman KV, McCall LM, et al. Factors associated with local-regional recurrence after a negative sentinel node dissection: results of the ACOSOG Z0010 trial. Ann Surg. 2012;256:428–36.
93. Nogi H, Uchida K, Mimoto R, et al. Long-term follow-up of node-negative breast cancer patients evaluated via sentinel node biopsy following neoadjuvant chemotherapy. Clin Breast Cancer. 2017;17:644. https://doi.org/10.1016/j.clbc.2017.05.002.
94. Balachandran VP, et al. Nomograms in oncology: more than meets the eye. Lancet Oncol. 2015;16(4):e173–80. https://doi.org/10.1016/S1470-2045(14)71116-7.
95. Hu X, Xue J, Peng S, et al. Preoperative nomogram for predicting sentinel lymph node metastasis risk in breast cancer: a potential application on omitting sentinel lymph node biopsy. Front Oncol. 2021;11:665240. https://doi.org/10.3389/fonc.2021.665240.
96. Tran HT, Pack D, Mylander C, et al. Ultrasound-based nomogram identifies breast cancer patients unlikely to harbor axillary metastasis: towards selective omission of sentinel lymph node biopsy. Ann Surg Oncol. 2020;27(8):2679–86. https://doi.org/10.1245/s10434-019-08164-3; Epub 2020 Feb 5.
97. Wang L, Li J, Qiao J, et al. Establishment of a model for predicting sentinel lymph node metastasis in early breast cancer based on contrast-enhanced ultrasound and clinicopathological features. Gland Surg. 2021;10(5):1701–12. https://doi.org/10.21037/gs-21-245.
98. Kuehn T, Bauerfeind I, Fehm T, et al. Sentinel-lymph-node biopsy in patients with breast cancer before and after neoadjuvant chemotherapy (SENTINA): a prospective, multicentre cohort study. Lancet Oncol. 2013;14(7):609–18. https://doi.org/10.1016/S1470-2045(13)70166-9.
99. Liedtke C, Kolberg HC, Kerschke L, et al. Systematic analysis of parameters predicting pathological axillary status (ypN0 vs. ypN) in patients with breast cancer converting from cN to ycN0 through primary systemic therapy (PST). Clin Exp Metastasis. 2018;35(8):777–83.

100. van Timmeren JE, Cester D, Tanadini-Lang S, et al. Radiomics in medical imaging-"how-to" guide and critical reflection. Insights Imaging. 2020;11(1):91. https://doi.org/10.1186/s13244-020-00887-2.
101. Zhou WJ, Zhang YD, Kong WT, et al. Preoperative prediction of axillary lymph node metastasis in patients with breast cancer based on radiomics of gray-scale ultrasonography. Gland Surg. 2021;10(6):1989–2001. https://doi.org/10.21037/gs-21-315.
102. Yu FH, Wang JX, Ye XH, et al. Ultrasound-based radiomics nomogram: a potential biomarker to predict axillary lymph node metastasis in early-stage invasive breast cancer. Eur J Radiol. 2019;119:108658. https://doi.org/10.1016/j.ejrad.2019.108658; Epub 2019 Sep 7.
103. Cyr AE, Tucker N, Ademuyiwa F, et al. Successful completion of the pilot phase of a randomized controlled trial comparing sentinel lymph node biopsy to no further axillary staging in patients with clinical T1-T2 N0 breast cancer and normal axillary ultrasound. J Am Coll Surg. 2016;223(2):399–407. https://doi.org/10.1016/j.jamcollsurg.2016.04.048; Epub 2016 May 20.
104. Gentilini O, Veronesi U. Abandoning sentinel lymph node biopsy in early breast cancer? A new trial in progress at the European Institute of Oncology of Milan (SOUND: sentinel node vs observation after axillary UltraSouND). Breast. 2012;21(5):678–81. https://doi.org/10.1016/j.breast.2012.06.013; Epub 2012 Jul 25.
105. Hildebrandt G, Stachs A, Gerber B, et al. Central review of radiation therapy planning among patients with breast-conserving surgery: results from a quality assurance process integrated into the INSEMA trial. Int J Radiat Oncol Biol Phys. 2020;107(4):683–93. https://doi.org/10.1016/j.ijrobp.2020.04.042; Epub 2020 May 11.
106. van Roozendaal LM, Vane MLG, van Dalen T, et al. Clinically node negative breast cancer patients undergoing breast conserving therapy, sentinel lymph node procedure versus follow-up: a Dutch randomized controlled multicentre trial (BOOG 2013-08). BMC Cancer. 2017;17(1):459. https://doi.org/10.1186/s12885-017-3443-x.

Validation Trials of Sentinel Node Biopsy in Breast Cancer

4

Basila A. Ali and Nita S. Nair

4.1 Introduction

Bartholin was the first to report on lymphatic system, and subsequently Virchow Virchow hypothesised that lymph nodes filter particulate matter. This led to the Halstedian era of en bloc radical surgery [1], which was then challenged by Fisher's theory that breast cancer is a systemic disease at presentation. Fisher proposed that involvement of lymph nodes was a hallmark of distant/systemic disease [2].

The present management of breast cancer is based on the spectrum theory proposing that breast cancer is best thought of as a spectrum of disease with increasing inclination towards metastasising as a function of tumour growth and progression [2]. As metastatic spread to the axillary lymph nodes follows a step ladder pattern, staging the axilla with conservative methods to avoid the morbidity of axillary lymph node dissection (ALND) was a logical step forward.

In 1977, Ramon Cabañas, a urologist, first described sentinel lymph node biopsy for penile carcinoma. In the late 1980s, Donald L. Morton and Alistair J. Cochran proposed the innovative concept of "lymphatic mapping with sentinel lymph node biopsy" for melanoma. They demonstrated that the first node that would receive lymphatic drainage from the tumour would depend on the site of the primary tumour and with individual variability [1].

B. A. Ali
Breast Surgical Oncology, Tata Memorial Centre, Homi Bhabha National Institute, Mumbai, Maharashtra, India

N. S. Nair (✉)
Department of Surgical Oncology, Breast Service, Tata Memorial Centre, Homi Bhabha National Institute, Mumbai, Maharashtra, India

Chintamani (ed.), *Sentinel Node Biopsy in Breast Cancer*,
https://doi.org/10.1007/978-81-322-3994-9_4

4.2 Sentinel Lymph Node (SLN) Biopsy: Initially Reported Studies on Breast Cancer

Axillary lymph node involvement is one of the most important prognostic factors in breast cancer [3]. There have been multiple attempts to stage the axilla accurately by clinical examination, ultrasound, magnetic resonance imaging, and positron emission tomography, which have not proven to be reliable. Staging the axilla by surgery continues to remain the gold standard in clinically N0 patients. Numerous authors described direct localisation of sentinel nodes (SLN) with the use of multiple dyes and hand-held devices [4, 5].

The first article of blue dye mapping in breast cancer was published by Guiliano in 1994 [6]. A total of 174 women underwent SLN using a vital dye injected at the primary breast cancer site. Axillary lymphatics were identified and followed to the first echelon node. This was first excised and analysed separately, and then ALND was completed. The identification rate of SLN was 65.5% (114/174), and it accurately predicted the axilla in 95.6% of women (109/114). The authors also reported that there was a definite learning curve, as false-negative SLN was mostly identified in the early part of the study. Additionally they reported that in the 54 evaluated for the location of SLN, 10 were identified in level 2 of the axilla.

Taking these findings forward, Krag et al. [7] reported on a cohort from 11 centres with 443 women with breast cancer. Technetium-99 m sulphur colloid (1 mCi [37 MBq]), 4 mL was injected into the breast around the tumour or biopsy cavity to identify hot spots in the axilla, representing SLN, which were identified using hand-held gamma probe. All patients underwent an ALND for validation of SLN. The overall identification rate of SLN was 93% (413 of 443 patients), and the accuracy was 97% (392 of 405). However, this method was associated with some technical issues and had a steeper learning curve.

These studies, however, paved the way for larger validation studies which now form the basis of our current practice and recommendations.

4.3 Validation of SLNB in Breast Cancer (Tables 4.1 and 4.2)

4.3.1 Understanding the Validation of SLN

The SLN is the first lymph node to which the primary tumour metastasises.

- Validation endpoints:
  - Identification rates/failure of procedure
  - False-negative rate/ability to predict the rest of the axilla
  - Regional recurrence/survival
  - Morbidity

Table 4.1 Landmark trials in the validation of SLN in breast cancer

Trial/author	Place	Total number of patients	Number of patients in the SLNB arm	Number of patients in the axillary dissection arm	Primary end points	Secondary end points
NSABP B-32	USA and Canada	5611	2804	2807	Comparison of OS	Comparison of DFS, local recurrences, morbidity
Veronesi et al	Milan	516	257	259	Predictive power of the status of the SLNB	Quality of life, axillary recurrence, DFS and OS
ALMANAC	Cardiff, UK	1031	515	516	Comparison of arm and shoulder morbidity and quality of life	Comparison of axillary recurrence rate
SENTINELLA	Veneto, Italy	697	345	352	Comparison of disease-free survival	Comparison of overall survival, morbidity and quality of life
SNAC	AUS + NZ	1088	544	544	% increase in arm circumference	No. of patients who had ≥15% increase in arm volume

Table 4.2 Landmark trial results on SLN accuracy

Trial/author	Year	SLN identification %	Sensitivity %	False negativity %
NSABP B-32	2007	97.3	90.2	9.8
Veronesi et al.	2003	98.5	91.2	8.8
ALMANAC	2006	98.0	93.3	6.7
SENTINELLA	2008	95	83.3	16.7
SNAC	2009	94.0	94.5	7.6

1. *Identification rate (IR)*: Failure to identify the SLN results in failure of the procedure, thus needing complete standard axillary dissection. Kim et al. [8] reported IR ranging from 41% to 100%, with >50% of studies reporting a rate <90%. One the most important factors associated with lower identification rates is the mapping technique. Double-dye techniques with radioactive isotopes in combination with coloured dyes produced higher IR than single-dye techniques.

Other factors that impact the identification rate are obesity, tumour location and surgeons' learning curve [9].

2. *The false-negative rate (FNR)*: Lower FNR of SLN helps accurately map the axilla and reduce the risk of leaving behind positive non-sentinel lymph nodes. The pitfalls of SLN are risks of false-negative SLN, understaging the axilla and leaving behind disease and potentially increasing the risk of recurrence. FNR is measured by comparing the histology of the SLN with the remaining lymph nodes excised in ALND. The common causes of false-negative SLN are rerouting of lymphatic drainage due to tumour blockage, sampling error by the pathologist and learning curve of the surgeon. A false-negative rate between 5–10% is considered acceptable with a narrow 95% confidence interval. [10] An inverse correlation is observed between the FNR of SLN reported in numerous trails and both the number of patients included in the study ($r = -0.42$; $P < 0.01$) and the proportion of patients with successful SLN mapping ($r = -0.32$; $P = 0.009$) [8].

4.3.2 Landmark Trials

Mentioned below are some of the landmark trials validating SLN in early breast cancer.

4.3.2.1 The Milan Trial

Veronesi et al. randomised 516 women with T1N0 early breast cancer to SLN followed by ALND versus SLN alone.[11] The primary end point of this study was the predictive power of SLN, (% of SLN accurately identified positive axillary nodal disease). Additional end points were quality of life, axillary recurrence rate and disease-free and overall survival.

Technical Results

A hallmark of this study was the extensive pathological evaluation the SLN. For each node that was large enough to be cut, 15 pairs of frozen sections, each 4-μm thick, were cut at 50-μm intervals in each half of the node, amounting to about 60 sections per node. If residual tissue was left, additional pairs of sections were cut at 100-μm intervals until the lymph node had been sampled completely. One section in each pair of sections was stained with haematoxylin and eosin (H&E). If the result was ambiguous, the other section was stained for cytokeratins by means of a rapid method and stained for the monoclonal antibody MNF116. This was unlike the pathological evaluation of SLN in any other trial.

The rest of the lymph nodes removed in ALND were analysed by standard pathological evaluation. If a lymph node was larger than 5 mm, they were bisected, if they were less than or equal to 5 mm they were embedded without cutting and 3–6 sections per lymph node obtained at different levels 100–500 μm apart and stained with routine H&E.

In the validation group, 32.3% SLN were positive on pathology, and in the SLN-alone arm, 35.5% were positive on pathology and underwent ALND. In the ALND arm, 8.8%% (8/91) had false-negative SLN, of whom 2 had only micro-metastatic disease in a single node. The overall accuracy of the SLN in the validation arm was thus 96.9%, with 91.2% sensitivity and 100% specificity. The false-negative rate was 8.8%, and the negative predictive value was 95.4%.

Patients on the SLN-alone arm reported less pain, numbness and better arm mobility. They also had less arm swelling than those who underwent ALND.

After a follow-up of 79 months, OS and DFS were similar in both arms. The overall 10-year survival was 89.7% (95% CI: 85.5–93.8) in the ALND arm and 93.5% (95% CI: 90.3–96.8%) in the SLN arm [12].

4.3.2.2 National Surgical Adjuvant Breast and Bowel Project (NSABP) B-32

The National Surgical Adjuvant Breast and Bowel Project (NSABP) B-32 trial [13] was designed to evaluate the therapeutic outcomes of SLN compared with ALND. The primary endpoints of the B-32 trial were survival, regional control and morbidity. The NSABP B-32 trial randomised 5611 women with node-negative early breast cancer to two groups. The first with 2807 women had SLN followed by ALND (the validation arm). The second with 2804 women underwent SLN, those with positive SLN underwent ALND, and those with negative SLN underwent observation of the remaining axilla.

The technical results [14] were reported in 5536 patients, with successful identification of SLN in 97.2% in the two groups. Identification of a pre-incision hot spot was associated with higher identification rate (98.9%). Overall, 1.4% of SLN were identified outside of axillary levels I and II. A small number of SLN (3.9%) were identified by palpation alone, and 65.1% were radioactive and blue. In the validation cohort, the accuracy of SLN was 97.1% with a false-negative rate of 9.8%. Differences in tumour location, type of biopsy and number of SLNs removed significantly affected the false-negative rate. Only 0.7% reported allergic reactions related to blue dye.

Morbidity related to range of motion, oedema, pain and sensory deficits was lower in the SLN-alone group compared with those who underwent ALND. Thus, the NSABP-B32 is recognised as a landmark trial that established the role of SLN as an accurate method to stage the axilla in clinically node-negative early breast cancer.

Training and Reducing FNR

This study also established rigorous training categories, after which the American Society of Breast Surgeons recommended that prior to offering SLN as standard practice, surgeons must demonstrate a rate of SLN identification of 85% with a false-negative rate of 5% or less in order to abandon axillary dissection [16].

Key Take-Home Messages: The NSABP B32 Trial Changed the Landscape of Sentinel Lymph Node Biopsy in Breast Cancer

Other than establishing the technical aspects and oncological safety of the SLNB procedure, this trial offered certain key concepts in the approach to SLN:

- Identification of pre-incision hot spot to improve success of the SLN technique.
- Only 1.4% SLN were located outside axillary levels I and II.
- After this study the definition of SLN included large palpable LN in addition to blue and hot nodes, as 3.9% of all SLN were identified by palpation alone.
- Role of occult metastasis, need for routine IHC or extensive sectioning was questioned. Occult metastasis was identified in 15.9% of cases. The 5 year-overall survival was 95.8% for patients who were lymph node-negative and 94.6% for those with occult lymph node metastasis ($p = 0.03$). The magnitude of the difference was small and not considered clinically significant, and thus extensive pathological evaluation was abandoned [17].

4.3.2.3 SENTINELLA/GIVOM [18]

The SENTINELLA trial randomised 697 patients to SLNB arm with ALND alone if the SLNB was positive and SLNB followed by ALND. The primary end point was disease free survival, and the secondary end points were overall survival, physical morbidity and quality of life comparisons. However this study accrual suffered as SLNB gained popularity and patients opted for SLN. The trial was designed as a noninferiority trial requiring a sample size of 1498 cases to demonstrate that the 5-year DFS for patients treated in the SLN arm was no worse than that in the ALND arm; however only 749 patients were accrued.

Technical Findings

For the 749 patients who were randomised, the authors reported an identification rate of 95% and false-negative rate of 16.7% (18 of 108) in the ALND arm. At a median follow-up of 56 months, the 5-year disease-free survival was 89.9% in the ALND arm compared with 87.6% in the SLN arm, with a difference of 2.3% (95% CI: −3.1% to 7.6%). However, as the number of enrolled patients was not sufficient, the authors were unable to draw any definitive conclusions.

Key Take Home Messages

- This study had an unusually high FNR of 16.7%, which was explained by the fact that this trial did not request a formal training course or a surgical quality control on site.
- The high false-negative rate did not seem to have a negative impact on outcomes. In the SLN arm, there were 4 recurrences, one in the axilla and 3 in the supraclavicular fossa.

4.3.2.4 The Axillary Lymph Mapping Against Nodal Axillary Clearance (ALMANAC) Trial

The aforementioned studies were all designed to validate SLN as a method to accurately stage the axilla in patients with clinically node-negative (cN0) early breast cancer. The ALMANAC trial [19] was designed with the primary end point of quality of life related to SLN compared with ALND. Patients with cN0 early breast cancer were randomised to SLN or ALND, and quality of life measures like lymphedema, shoulder morbidity and sensory loss were evaluated.

Technical Findings

The identification rate of SLN was 96.1%. Factors associated with failure to localise SLN were obesity ($p < 0.001$), tumour location ($p = 0.008$) and non-pre-incision hot spot identified ($p < 0.001$). The median number of SLN removed per patient was 2 (range 1–9). FNR was lower with more number of nodes removed, 10.1% in those with one SLN compared with 1.1% in those who had multiple SLNs (three or more) removed ($p = 0.010$) [9].

Patients in the SLNB group reported lower incidence of lymphoedema of 5% compared with 13% in ALND (RR 0.37). At 12 months sensory loss in the distribution of the intercostobrachial nerve was also less in the SLNB group than in the ALND group (11% vs 31%, respectively) (RR 0.37). Finally shoulder function was significantly impaired in the ALND group at 1 month, with no long-term detriment noted on follow-up. Quality of life was assessed using the FACT-B + 4 questionnaires (Functional Assessment of Cancer Therapy-Breast) which favoured the SLNB group.

On follow-up, axillary nodal metastases were higher in the SLN arm (26% vs 23%; difference = 2.4%, 95% CI = −3.0% to 7.7%) [19].

Key Take Away Points

- This trial included male patients, had no restriction on tumour size and type of surgery comprising of both breast conservation surgery and mastectomy.
- This study did not have intraoperative pathological diagnosis, and SLNB was evaluated at final histopathology, thus needing a secondary procedure if the lymph nodes were positive.
- The significant difference in lymphoedema rates reported i.e. 5% versus 13% at 12 months; between SLN and ALND arms were patient reported outcomes.

4.3.2.5 RACS Sentinel Node Biopsy Versus Axillary Clearance (SNAC) 1 Trial [20]

The SNAC trial (sentinel node biopsy vs axillary clearance), another randomised trial evaluating morbidity of SLN compared with ALND, randomised 1088 patients to SNLB and axillary dissection (only if SLNB was positive or not identified) and ALND. The primary end point was percentage increase in arm volume.

Technical Results

The average increases in arm volume in SLNB and ALND at 6–12 months were 2.8% and 4.2%, respectively. There was thus a 1.4% increase reported in the ALND group. The number of patients who had an increase in arm volume of 15% or more from baseline was 4.2% in the SLNB arm compared with 6.9% in the ALND arm.

Updated results at 5-year follow reported arm volume progressively in the ALND and SLN arms up to 2 years and accompanied by weight gain. Factors associated with increased risk of lymphoedema were surgery type (ALND vs SLN), obesity, diabetes, palpable tumour and weight gain on follow-up exceeding 10% of baseline [21].

References

1. Tanis PJ, Nieweg OE, Valdés Olmos RA, et al. History of sentinel node and validation of the technique. Breast Cancer Res. 2001;3:109–12.
2. Hellman S. Natural history of small breast cancers. J Clin Oncol. 1994;12:2229–34.
3. Carter CL, Allen C, Henson DE. Relation of tumor size, lymph node status, and survival in 24,740 breast cancer cases. Cancer. 1989;63:181–7.
4. Haagensen CD, Feind KR, Herter FP, Slanetz CA, Weinberg JA. The lymphatics in cancer. Philadelphia: WB Saunders Company; 1972.
5. Krag DN, Weaver DL, Alex JC, Fairbank JT. Surgical resection and radiolocalization of the sentinel lymph node in breast cancer using a gamma probe. Surg Oncol. 1993;2:335–9.
6. Giuliano AE, Kirgan DM, Guenther JM, Morton DL. Lymphatic mapping and sentinel lymphadenectomy for breast cancer. Ann Surg. 1994;220:391–8.
7. Krag D, Weaver D, Ashikaga T, et al. The sentinel node in breast cancer — a multicenter validation study. N Engl J Med. 1998;339:941–6.
8. Kim T, Giuliano AE, Lyman GH. Lymphatic mapping and sentinel lymph node biopsy in early-stage breast carcinoma: a metaanalysis. Cancer. 2006;106(1):4–16.
9. Goyal A, Newcombe RG, Chhabra A, Mansel RE, ALMANAC Trialists Group. Factors affecting failed localisation and false-negative rates of sentinel node biopsy in breast cancer--results of the ALMANAC validation phase. Breast Cancer Res Treat. 2006;99(2):203–8.
10. Tanis PJ, Nieweg OE, Hart AA, Kroon BB. The illusion of the learning phase for lymphatic mapping. Ann Surg Oncol. 2002;9(2):142–7.
11. Veronesi U, Paganelli G, Viale G, et al. randomized comparison of sentinel-node biopsy with routine axillary dissection in breast cancer. N Engl J Med. 2003;349(6):546–53.
12. Veronesi U, Viale G, Paganelli G, et al. Sentinel lymph node biopsy in breast cancer. Ann Surg. 2010;251(4):595–600.
13. Krag DN, Anderson SJ, Julian TB. Sentinel-lymph-node resection compared with conventional axillary-lymph-node dissection in clinically node-negative patients with breast cancer: overall survival findings from the NSABP B-32 randomised phase 3 trial. Lancet Oncol. 2010;11(10):927–33.
14. Krag DN, Anderson SJ, Julian TB, et al. National Surgical Adjuvant Breast and Bowel Project. Technical outcomes of sentinel-lymph-node resection and conventional axillary-lymph-node dissection in patients with clinically node-negative breast cancer: results from the NSABP B-32 randomised phase III trial. Lancet Oncol. 2007;8(10):881–8.
15. Krag DN, Ashikaga T, Harlow SP, Skelly JM, Julian TB, Brown AM, Weaver DL, Wolmark N. National Surgical Adjuvant Breast and Bowel Project. Surgeon training, protocol compliance, and technical outcomes from breast cancer sentinel lymph node randomized trial. J Natl Cancer Inst. 2009;101(19):1356–62.
16. Lyman GH, Giuliano AE, Somerfield MR, et al. American Society of Clinical Oncology guideline recommendations for sentinel lymph node biopsy in early-stage breast cancer. J Clin Oncol. 2005;23(30):7703–20.
17. Wu Y, Mittendorf EA, Kelten C, et al. Occult axillary lymph node metastases do not have prognostic significance in early stage breast cancer. Cancer. 2012;118:1507–14.
18. Zavagno G, De Salvo GL, Scalco GIVOM, Trialists. A Randomized clinical trial on sentinel lymph node biopsy versus axillary lymph node dissection in breast cancer: results of the Sentinella/GIVOM trial. Ann Surg. 2008;247(2):207–13.
19. Mansel RE, Fallowfield L, Kissin M, et al. Randomized multicenter trial of sentinel node biopsy versus standard axillary treatment in operable breast cancer: the ALMANAC Trial. J Natl Cancer Inst. 2006;98(9):599–609.

20. Gill G, SNAC Trial Group of the Royal Australasian College of Surgeons (RACS) and NHMRC Clinical Trials Centre. Sentinel-lymph-node-based management or routine axillary clearance? One-year outcomes of sentinel node biopsy versus axillary clearance (SNAC): a randomized controlled surgical trial. Ann Surg Oncol. 2009;16(2):266–75.
21. Wetzig N, Gill PG, Espinoza D, et al. Sentinel-lymph-node-based management or routine axillary clearance? Five-year outcomes of the RACS sentinel node biopsy versus axillary clearance (SNAC) 1 trial: assessment and incidence of true lymphedema. Ann Surg Oncol. 2017;24(4):1064–70.

5 Sentinel Lymph Node Biopsy in Breast Cancer-Techniques

Chintamani and Sukriti Rastogi

The involvement of axillary lymph nodes in breast cancer generally indicates poor prognosis with an associated drop in 5-year survival rates by 28–40%. Until the 1980s, axillary lymph node dissection (ALND) was considered the gold standard in managing the axilla while treating and staging breast cancer and also for planning adjuvant therapy. Based on the understanding that tumour cells migrate in an orderly and predictable manner from the primary site to the first echelon lymph nodes (sentinel nodes) before draining into subsequent nodes, there has been a paradigm shift toward de-escalation in addressing the axilla without compromising the oncological outcomes.

Non-invasive staging of the axilla is usually not optimum. Physical examination does not accurately predict lymph node involvement and has a false-negative rate (FNR) of up to 45% [1]. In clinically node-negative (cNo) axilla, even imaging modalities such as ultrasonography, magnetic resonance imaging, and positron emission tomography/computed tomography have proven to be of limited value in staging the axilla accurately [2–4]. Consequently, to predict the status of the axilla and avoid potentially morbid ALND, the role of SNLB has evolved (NSABP-32 trial etc.) and is currently being established as the standard of care in clinically and sonologically node-negative axilla.

Krag et al. pioneered the technique of sentinel lymph node biopsy in breast cancer by radio-localisation via peri-tumoural injection of technetium 99m (99mTc) sulphur colloid. They reported an 82% ($n = 22$) identification rate (IR) with a 100%

Chintamani (✉)
Chief-Breast and Endocrine Unit, Department of Surgery Vardhman Mahavir Medical College Safdarjang Hospital, New Delhi, New Delhi, India

Breast and Endocrine Unit, Department of Surgery, Vardhman Mahavir Medical College, Safdarjang Hospital, New Delhi, New Delhi, India

S. Rastogi
Chief-Breast and Endocrine Unit ,Department of Surgery Vardhman Mahavir Medical College Safdarjang Hospital, New Delhi, New Delhi, India

Chintamani (ed.), *Sentinel Node Biopsy in Breast Cancer*,
https://doi.org/10.1007/978-81-322-3994-9_5

accuracy in predicting axillary node status [5]. It was followed by intra-operative vital blue dye mapping by Giuliano et al. who reported an IR of 65% with a sensitivity of 88% and 6.5% false-negative results [6]. Albertini et al. were the first to combine these two techniques and successfully detected sentinel nodes (SNs) in 92% of cases ($n = 62$) with 100% predictive accuracy [7].

There are various methods used to map the sentinel lymph nodes, and this is one of the most critical factors affecting the IRs and FNRs of SLNB, and to date, there is no standardised protocol for performing this procedure. There are various methods of doing it, and newer ones are emerging. However, irrespective of the technique, a sentinel lymph node can still be identified in approximately 96% of the patients, and that is good news [7, 8].

Many studies report a higher IR with the combined usage of blue dye and radioisotope techniques, which is considered more reliable and superior to the use of a single method in isolation [9–11]. The IRs were 96–97% in the ALMANAC trials with the dual technique [12], which is now considered the gold standard for SLNB. These two methods are complementary, with blue dye providing additional visual guidance that simplifies the procedure.

The section below describes the commonly used tracer agents in SLNB:

1. Blue dye
2. Radioactive colloid

5.1 Blue Dye

The ideal blue dye for SLNB should have the highest IR and the lowest adverse effect rates. The most commonly used blue dyes are isosulfan blue (1%), patent blue V sodium (2.5%) and methylene blue dye (MBD) (1%) (MBD). Blue dyes have different molecular structures, which give them unique characteristics. Isosulfan and patent blue show high protein affinity due to sulfonic acids. They combine with amino groups on the protein surface, while MBD shows no protein affinity at 37 °C.

5.1.1 Isosulfan Blue

Also known as Lymphazurin blue, isosulfan blue is an isomer of patent blue V which has calcium- and sodium-based salt. The latter is used in SLNB as it binds to albumin and other proteins to get absorbed by the lymphatic system.

5.1.2 Patent Blue V

It is known by various names such as Alphazurine, sulfan blue, sulfane blue, patent blue violet and patent blue pure. It has a similar mechanism of action to isosulfan blue.

5.1.3 Methylene Blue

Koller first reported the use of methylene blue for SLNB. It is a dark green crystalline compound that becomes dark blue in solution. Besides having a diagnostic role in SLNB, Barrett's oesophagus, urinary fistulae, parathyroids, etc., it also has a therapeutic role in resuscitation to improve outcomes in patients with hypovolemic shock [13]. Due to its wider availability, no potential life-threatening allergic reactions and lower cost, many centres (including the author) prefer using MBD alone. It is safe even for pregnant patients and is an effective alternative to isosulfan and patent blue.

In a systematic review by Li J et al. [14], 18 studies were included that used MBD alone for SLNB, and they showed an IR of 91%, FNR of 13%, pooled sensitivity of 87%, NPV of 91%, and accuracy rate of 94%. Han C et al. [15] conducted a mini-review on factors with false-negative sentinel lymph node biopsies in breast cancer with MBD alone. They found that smaller tumour volume, increased number of SNs, removal of any large or hard LNs and improved surgeon experience can lower FNR. Studies have found methylene blue to be superior to other blue dyes with respect to FNRs. However, there was no significant difference in IRs after adding two random effects during statistical analysis [16].

To abandon axillary dissection, the American Society of Breast Surgeons recommends an IR of 85% and an FNR of 5% or less [17].

Adverse events associated with blue dye include interference with pulse oximetry, tattooing of the skin, discoloration of body fluids and anaphylactic and allergic reactions, which are usually severe with isosulfan blue, requiring resuscitation in 0.16–1.1% of cases [17–20].

A skin test to detect any hypersensitivity may be performed, but it lacks sensitivity. Routine prophylaxis is not recommended. But in high-risk cases, the severity and not the incidence of hypersensitivity reaction can be reduced with prophylactic treatment using 100 mg of hydrocortisone (or 20 mg of methylprednisolone or 4 mg of dexamethasone), 50 mg of diphenhydramine, and 20 mg of famotidine intravenously just before or at the time of induction [18].

Methylene blue has lower rates of anaphylactic reactions (0.0006%) [20–22]. But it does have some other side effects, like intradermal injection, which can lead to skin necrosis, and intraparenchymal injection, which can cause induration, pain and erythema in some cases [23]. There are reports of patients on serotonergic medications developing pulmonary oedema and serotonin syndrome with MBD [24]. These side effects can potentially be minimised by diluting methylene blue with normal saline at a ratio of 1:1 to 1:7 [25].

5.2 Radioactive Colloid

Several colloidal radioisotopes that are used for SLN mapping include filtered and unfiltered technetium-99m sulphur colloid, technetium-99m tin (antimony) colloid, technetium-99m labelled albumin nanocolloid, Tc-99m-pertechnetate and

Tc-99m-dextran. The success rates of SLN detection is mainly determined by the particle size and surface characteristics of the colloidal particles, which influence the rate of migration of the agent from the injection site to the lymphatic capillaries and its phagocytosis by lymph node macrophages. The aim is, therefore, rapid transport of the colloid particles to the SLN with persistent retention.

The unfiltered radioactive colloid is better for SLNB because larger particles (100–1000 nm) in the unfiltered solution are trapped better and for longer time period by the sentinel lymph nodes which could lower the FNRs. By contrast, the filtered colloid is better for lymphoscintigraphy as the smaller colloidal particles have a faster lymphatic drainage from the injection site, enabling faster imaging of the SLNs before passing onto the second and third echelon nodes in the axilla. However, particles smaller than 5 nm are not ideal because they get cleared from the injection site through the lymphatics and blood capillaries.

Newer and more effective radiotracers are being developed, for example 99mTc-tilmanocept (99mTc-TM), which has more rapid clearance from the injection site, higher degree of localisation and SLN extraction rates and lower distal node accumulation than Tc-99m-colloidal albumin but similar SLN uptake as 99mTc-sulphur colloid.

99mTc-rituximab developed by Li et al. contains 99mTc-labeled monoclonal antibody targeting CD20 expressed abundantly on the surface of B-cells in LNs. Its uniform molecular weight and size prevent its migration from sentinel to the second echelon LNs, achieving clear SLN imaging and higher success rates of lymphoscintigraphy [26].

Recently, İlem-Özdemir et al. prepared a novel combination of RI and BD called 99mTc-isosulfan blue to be used as a single agent but is still under evaluation. Its effectiveness in mapping LNs has been examined in rats and has shown promising results [27].

The availability of nuclear medicine facilities, trained staff and specialised handling and disposal of isotopes pose logistic challenges to the use of radioactive colloid. Therefore, the institution must establish the safeguards for using radioactive materials and their disposal. Preparation and injection of the radiocolloid agent as well as careful and appropriate disposal of radioactively contaminated equipment and gloves should take place under the auspices of an approved nuclear medicine department. It also causes a low level of radiation exposure both to the patients and healthcare staff. Some patients may even be reluctant, so obtaining informed consent is mandatory. Random radiation monitoring of the areas that may be exposed to radioactive contamination should be performed. However, in the operating rooms, additional shielding, monitoring devices or particular trash disposal protocols are not required.

5.3 Sentinel Lymph Node Biopsy: The Technique

Clinical practices vary regarding the injection techniques for SLNB. It is mainly related to the lymphatic drainage pattern of the breast and of the tumour, which, regardless of the location, drains through a common afferent lymphatic channel to a common axillary sentinel lymph node explaining the identification of the same lymph nodes irrespective of the site of injection.

5.3.1 Sites of Injection

5.3.1.1 Intradermal, Intraparenchymal and Sub-areolar

Various sites for injecting radiocolloids and dyes are the *peri-tumoural, periareolar or sub-areolar* regions (Fig. 5.1), through the *intradermal, subdermal or intraparenchymal routes*, respectively.

Nieweg classified the injection sites for sentinel node biopsy (SLN) mapping in breast into two categories: deep (peri-tumoural, subtumoural and intratumoural) and superficial (intradermal, subdermal, periareolar and sub-areolar) [28].

A study conducted by Sappey using dual-tracer injection confirmed that the sub-areolar lymphatic plexus (Sappey's plexus), the dermis of the skin, and breast parenchyma have a common embryological origin and drainage pattern to the same axillary nodes [29]. This formed the basis for superficial (intradermal, subdermal) and central (sub-areolar, periareolar) injections.

Initially, deep peri-tumoural, tracer administration was preferred over superficial sites and was much promoted by the northern European teams that observed an SLN IR of 97.2% and an FNR of 3.1% [30]. Giuliano et al. [31] and Cox et al. [32] strongly advocated the use of intraparenchymal injection, supported by the results of 1% or less FNRs and near 100% IRs. However, this approach has been criticised based on its limited role in non-palpable, multi-centric tumours and upper outer

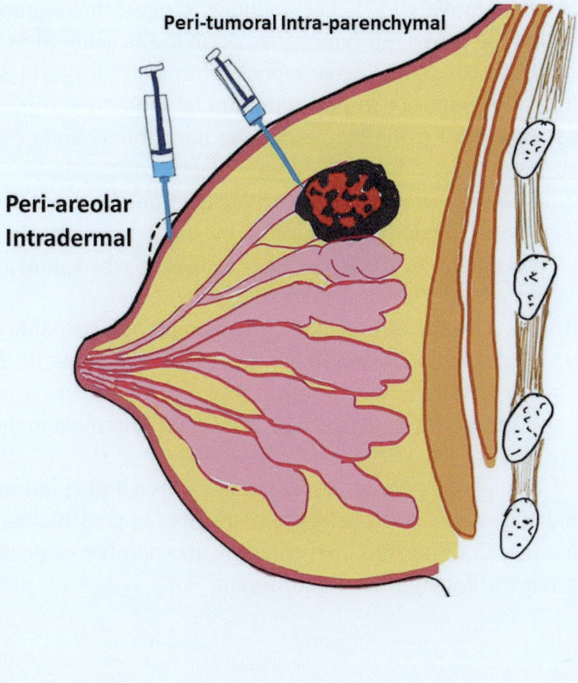

Fig. 5.1 Periareolar intradermal injection of blue dye. The needle is inserted at an acute angle and the bleb forms when the dye is injected

quadrant lesions due to the 'shine through phenomenon', i.e., overlapping signals from the injection site and the axilla. Peri-tumoural injection has another disadvantage of requiring considerable experience to achieve higher success rates of SLNB, as injecting the tracer correctly into the peri-tumoural parenchyma to a depth like that of the lesion is technically difficult. Also, one should be careful not to inject the dye into the tumour because tumour cells may impede the lymphatics or into the seroma cavity after breast biopsy as the seroma does not contain lymphatic channels. These errors in the technique may result in failures.

Sub-areolar injection of blue dye was first reported by Kern with a 98% IR and 0% FNR in 40 patients and is found to be a simpler and safer method that does not require extensive expertise with similar results when compared to peri-tumoural or intraparenchymal dye injections [33].

Veronesi et al. successfully reported an IR of 98% (n = 163) and FNR of 5.4% using a gamma probe after subdermal injection of 99mTc-colloidal albumin [34].

Jiyu Li et al. observed that the IRs for SLNB in studies using sub-areolar injection (94%) were significantly higher than those in studies using peri-tumoural injection (89%) [14].

Borgstein et al. injected the blue dye subdermally over the primary tumour in 90 cases and into the periareolar region in 130 procedures and observed 94% concordance between the two techniques [8].

Rodier et al. also reported similar IRs in both the periareolar and peri-tumoural injection groups [35].

Another study by Borgstein et al. on 220 patients comparing periareolar blue dye with peri-tumoural radiocolloid demonstrated that all blue nodes were hot [36]. Similarly, the non-randomised study of Bauer compared peri-tumoural and sub-areolar injections with both blue dye and radioisotope and reported 95% and 97% IRs, respectively [37]. These studies suggest that regardless of the tumour location within the breast, all lymphatics drain to the same SLN.

However, studies have reported intradermal (periareolar) injection of radiocolloid to be superior to peri-tumoural or subdermal injection [38]. There are several advantages of using the periareolar injection technique over others:

1. It does not require an accurate injection site and is relatively easier to perform.
2. Due to the dense sub-areolar plexus, which rapidly clears the tracer agents, its percentage to reach the SLN is higher when injected via the periareolar route than the peri-tumoural route.
3. It is a useful approach in patients with non-palpable and multicentric tumours.
4. For tumours located in the outer upper quadrant of the breast, periareolar injection increases the distance between the injection site and axillary SLN, thus reducing the shine-through effect and improved identification of SLNs.

Though the periareolar injection yields a higher number of sentinel lymph nodes, the purpose is not to detect as many SNs as possible but to identify the node that is the first draining site. Nevertheless, the number of positive nodes detected in both groups is not significantly different.

Extra-axillary sentinel nodes (EASN) or internal mammary (IM) nodes are usually associated with medial quadrant tumours and are more likely to be visualised after peri-tumoural injection [39–42]. However, they are not routinely dissected by most surgeons [43].

5.4 Dosage

5.4.1 Blue Dye

The most commonly used doses of blue dye (1% isosulfan blue or diluted methylene blue) for SNB are 2 ml and 5 ml. In a systematic review of 18 studies by Li J et al., the volume of MBD varied from 0.1 ml to 10 ml, and no difference was observed in the IR or FNR between 2-ml and 5-ml injections of MBD [14]. In elderly patients (above 65 years) or in patients with large breasts, one can consider increasing the injection volume to 8–10 cc due to a higher risk of failure to map the SLNs.

5.4.2 Radioactive Colloid

The amount of radioactive colloid to be injected depends on the duration between the administration of the tracer and the initiation of SLNB, and the optimal interval between both still needs to be determined. However, as suggested by previous studies, it varies from 30 min to 24 h [7, 8, 44–47].

5.4.3 1-Day Protocol (Interval of 1–6 h)

The most commonly used dosage is 0.5 mCi of Tc-99m-labeled radiopharmaceutical in a volume of 0.2 ml intradermally or 4–8 ml peri-tumourally. The nuclear medicine technologist carries the radioisotope in a lead case to the operating room for injection on the day of surgery.

5.4.4 2-Day Protocol (Interval of 16–20 h)

Tc-99m-labeled radiocolloid (2.5 mCi) is injected a day before surgery at a volume of 0.2 ml intradermally or 4–8 ml peri-tumourally. The 6-hour half-life of technetium sulphur colloid restricts the scheduling of surgery. Intratumoral injection requires higher volume and radioactivity to overcome the high intratumoral pressure and takes longer to visualise the SLNs.

No considerable difference in the number of SLNs harvested and the FNRs has been noted between the 1- and 2-day protocols. But, the 2-day protocol may have the advantages of high SLN-to-background and significantly low radioactivity in the resected specimen compared with the 1-day protocol. It allows efficient use of operating room time by avoiding delays imposed by injecting on the day of surgery. However, intra-operative radioisotope injection is more convenient, effective, safe, and comfortable for the patient.

5.5 Pre-operative Lymphoscintigraphy

SLNB was first performed widely in malignant melanoma. Considering variable lymphatic drainage, which may be far from the primary tumour site, pre-operative lymphoscintigraphy proves beneficial in these cases as it provides a wide field of view in locating SLNs. However, breast lymphatic drainage is relatively confined to the axilla, and studies have concluded that pre-operative lymphoscintigraphy is not a prerequisite for SLNB in breast cancer patients with the aspect of successful identification of SLN intra-operatively, especially with the dual-tracer technique. McMaster et al. [48] and Burak et al. [49] have reported no significant difference in FNRs between patients that underwent lymphoscintigraphy and those that did not. Moreover, the handheld gamma probe with a collimator has a narrow view field, and its sensitivity is still lower than the handheld gamma detector used intra-operatively [50]. In addition, pre-operative lymphoscintigraphy increases the cost and delays of surgery while making the patients more nervous pre-operatively.

5.6 Steps of SLNB

1. *Administering the tracer*
   (a) Radiocolloid and the blue dye are injected through the intra-/peri-tumoural route or the intra-/sub-dermal route over the tumour site or the peri-/sub-areolar route using a 25-G needle as discussed earlier (Figs. 5.2 and 5.3).
   (b) Air bubble (0.2 mL) is drawn into the syringe behind the radiocolloid to ensure that the whole amount is injected with minimal spillage, leaving none in the needle to avoid false results. Applying dry gauze at the injection site while the needle is being withdrawn is useful.

Fig. 5.2 Peri-tumoural injection site for the tracer

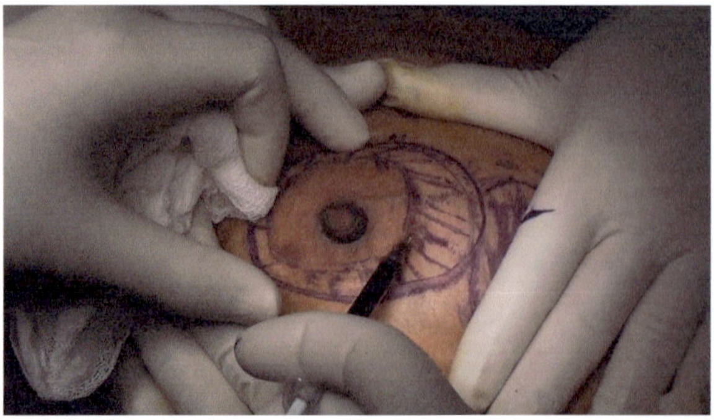

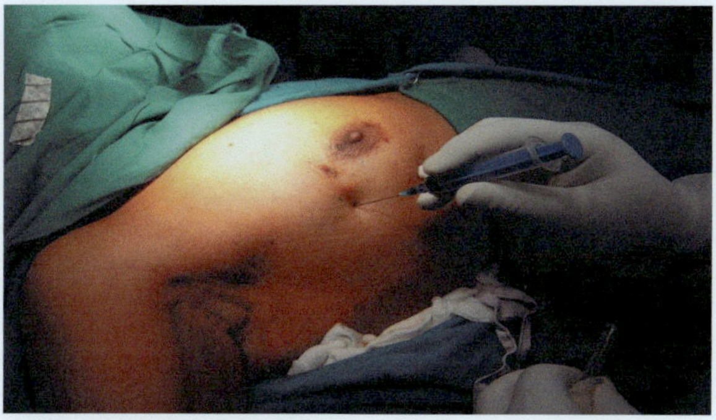

Fig. 5.3 Periareolar intradermal injection of the blue dye. The needle is inserted at an acute angle with the skin and the bleb forms when the dye is injected

(c) In peri-tumoural injection, the radiocolloid is injected deep into the breast parenchyma around the tumour at usually four sites, namely, superior, medial, inferior and lateral to the lump, or it may be injected in a semicircle along the axillary side of the lump. If the lesion is non-palpable, the needle is placed under ultrasound guidance.

(d) To inject intradermally, the needle is inserted at an acute angle to the skin, and a dermal skin wheal, or a bleb, is raised unlike in subdermal injection, which is performed beneath the skin into the subcutaneous tissue.

(e) Similarly, MBD is injected 5 min before making the incision, after which the breast is gently massaged for about 5 min to dilate breast lymphatics and accelerate the drainage of the tracer agent.

2. *Identifying radioactivity*

   A handheld gamma probe is used to identify the maximum radioactivity in the axilla. The camera should be equipped with a low-energy, high-resolution collimator and peaked at 140 KeV with a 20% window centred over the peak. In case one fails to locate a hotspot before incision, 10 to 40 mL of saline or local anaesthetic can be injected into the previous site of radioactive colloid injection, followed by repeat breast massage. This increases the interstitial pressure, forcing more tracer to drain into lymphatic channels. The risk of failure is higher in patients with a history of previous breast or axillary surgery due to blockage of normal lymphatic channels and formation of altered lymphatic drainage pathways. In such cases, pre-operative lymphoscintigraphy, along with the use of dual tracers, may be preferred.

3. *Making the incision*

   For SLNB, conventionally, an incision of about 2–3 cm is made in the hairline in the axilla and may be guided by the radiocolloid activity/ICG, depending on the modality adopted (Figs. 5.4 and 5.5).

   The incision for SLNB should be such that it can be extended or utilised for subsequent ALND when indicated.

4. *Identifying sentinel node*

   (a) After making the incision in the axillary fascia, one must carefully look for blue lymphatic channels, which, once identified, can be traced through gentle and ideally bloodless dissection to reach the sentinel lymph nodes (Figs. 5.6, 5.7, 5.8, 5.9, 5.10 and 5.11).

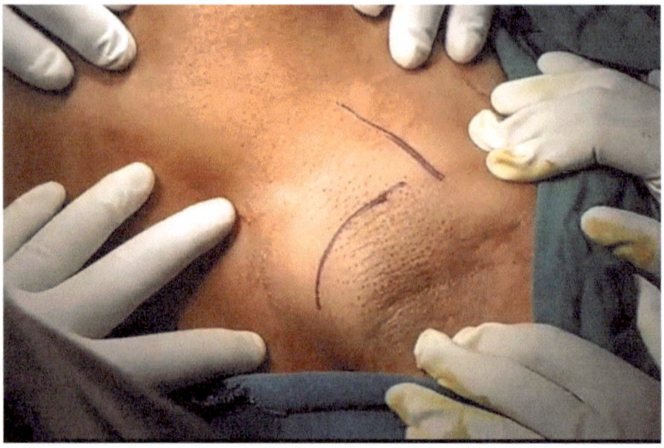

Fig. 5.4 Marking the incision for sentinel lymph node biopsy

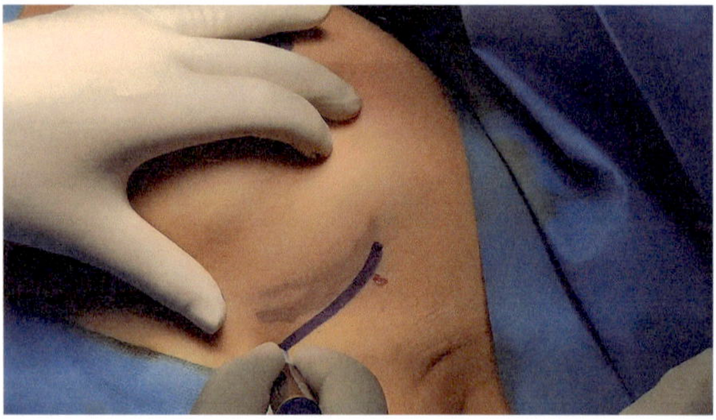

Fig. 5.5 Marking the incision for sentinel lymph node biopsy

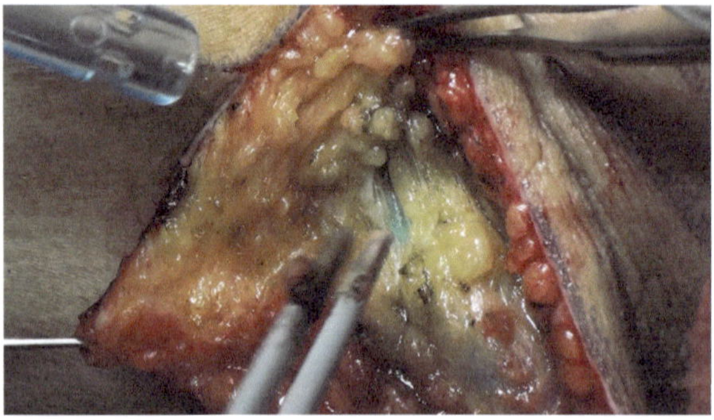

Fig. 5.6 Identifying and tracing the blue dye-stained lymphatic channel

(b) Blue nodes located most proximal to the tumour must be removed because staining of distal, non-sentinel lymph nodes may also happen with the rapid migration of the blue dye.
(c) Suspicious palpable nodes should also be removed for evaluation as a lymph node replaced with tumour is unlikely to take up the dye.
(d) The most radioactive lymph node detected by the gamma probe is removed first, and an ex vivo count is obtained. Removal of subsequent lymph nodes follows the "10 per cent rule," i.e. all lymph nodes with counts over 10% of the most radioactive node should be removed [51].

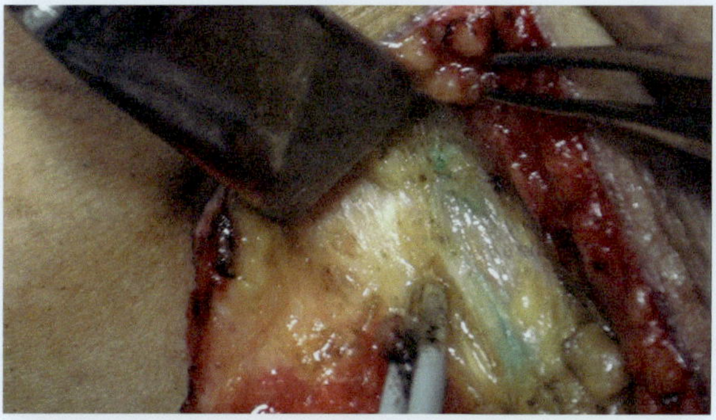

Fig. 5.7 Identifying and tracing the blue dye-stained lymphatic channel

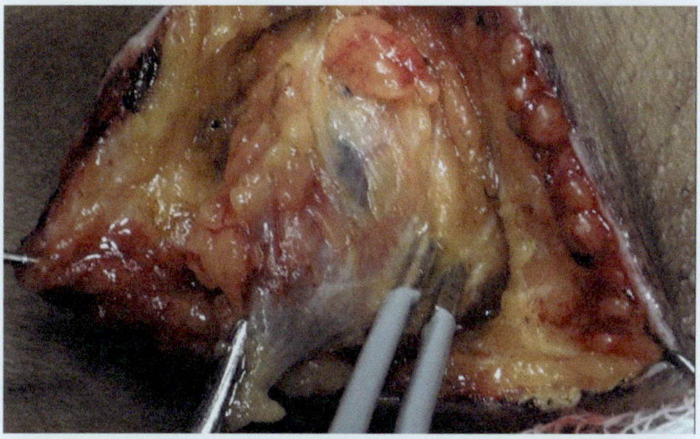

Fig. 5.8 Identifying the blue-coloured sentinel lymph node

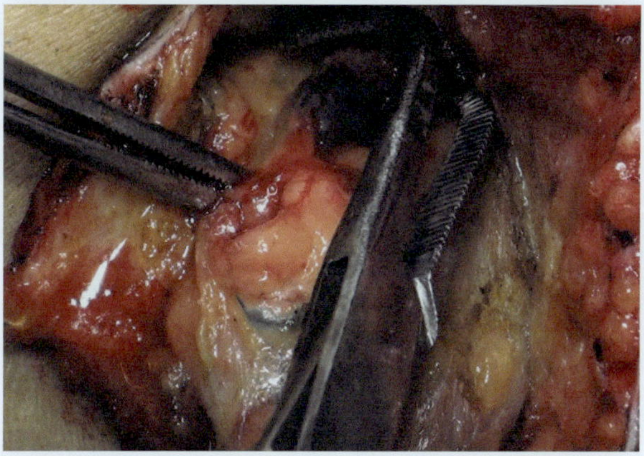

Fig. 5.9 Dissecting the sentinel lymph node

(e) Usually, two to three sentinel lymph nodes are removed [52]. Beyond four or five sentinel lymph nodes, the value of additional nodes is extremely low. Any suspicious palpable nodes should also be removed, regardless of whether they are radioactive since tumour-laden nodes may not take up much tracer.

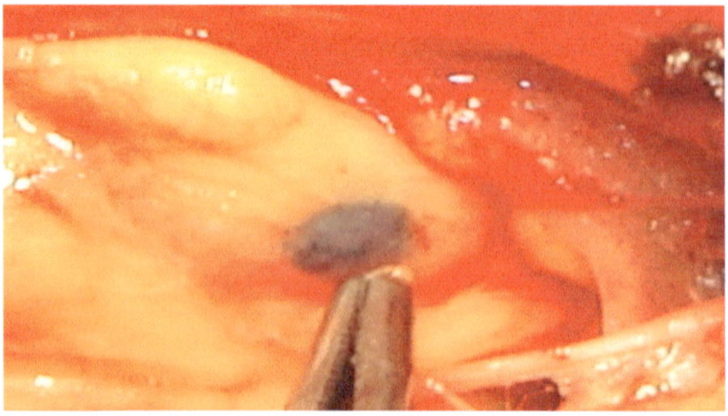

Fig. 5.10 Intra-operative photograph following injection of methylene blue showing blue lymphatic channels leading to a blue SLN

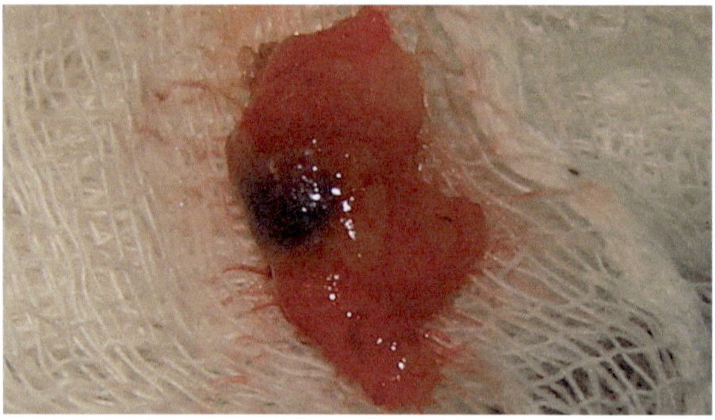

Fig. 5.11 Dissected specimen of blue SLN

(f) On completion, one must determine the background count and ex vivo radioactivity for every excised node using the gamma probe. In case of a 'high residual bed count' in the axilla, it is essential that all the 'hottest' nodes have been removed. If the remaining bed counts are uniform and remain over 10% with no 'discreet' areas of greater radioactivity found, then other nodes need not be removed unless they are suspicious by palpation.

5. *Pathological assessment of sentinel node*

Resected sentinel lymph nodes are taken in normal saline for a frozen section for metastasis.

Any tumour deposit in the axillary fat is typically classified as a 'positive node'. SN metastasis is grouped based on the size of the largest tumour deposit into the following:

(a) *Isolated tumour cell clusters*—small clusters of tumour cells not greater than 0.2 mm or non-confluent or nearly confluent clusters of cells not exceeding 200 cells in a single cross-section [53]. AJCC 8th edition defines isolated tumour cell clusters as pN0(i+) [54].
(b) *Micro-metastases*—metastatic deposit >0.2 mm but ≤2.0 mm. If present, it is designated as $pN1_{mi}$ according to the AJCC staging system.
(c) *Macro-metastases*—any tumour cell deposit >2.0 mm. It is classically designated as "node-positive".

Occult metastatic disease—nodal metastases that are not seen on initial haematoxylin and eosin examination but are detected subsequently on immunohistochemical staining or reverse transcriptase polymerase chain reaction (which is not recommended for routine evaluation). The occult micro-metastases have no significance in terms of surgical management and patient outcomes [55, 56].

Histologically negative nodes that are positive on immunohistochemistry staining or reverse transcriptase polymerase chain reaction are still classified as pN0 as per the AJCC 8th edition.

Extra-nodal extension (ENE) in SLNs, defined as the presence of tumour cells or clusters outside of the lymph node capsule, is associated with an increased burden of axillary lymph node metastasis with reported incidence ranging from 58 to 84% [57–59].

6. Primary tissue specimens obtained at surgery should be well marked with 'radioactive' labels and kept separated in areas designated for radioactive material for 72 h after injection of the radiopharmaceutical. After this time, they can be handled in the usual manner. Lymph nodes should also be kept separated for 36 h and marked with "radioactive" labels.

   One can prevent the 'shine-through' effect with tumours in the upper outer quadrant or axillary tail of the breast in the following ways:

   (a) Attaching a collimator to the gamma probe, making it more directional
   (b) Administering a smaller volume of the radioactive colloid that will limit the size of the diffusion zone, facilitating identification of axillary hotspots
   (c) Sub-areolar injection instead of peri-tumoural that will increase the distance between the injection site and axilla, minimising the potential for overlap

   These solutions would require the surgeon to anticipate the problem before injection. If the problem is discovered after injection, the surgeon should proceed with tumour resection, which eliminates the interference from the injection site when re-evaluating the axilla afterwards.

   Radiation Hazard to the Provider

   After the procedure, the surgeon's torso receives 1.33 mrem/h, the pathologist's torso receives 0.34 mrem/h, and the scrub nurse's torso receives 0.15 mrem/h. The surgeon's hands, receiving the maximum dose of radiation, would not exceed the maximum limit until they operate around 2190 h per year [60].

   Internal Mammary Nodes

   Removing radioactive internal mammary (IM) nodes is not recommended as it may not change the management and mostly if they are planned to be targeted during radiotherapy. According to Klauber-DeMoreÕs opinion [61], dissection of IM nodes has a minimal role based on the following reasons. First, IM SLNB would affect systemic therapy in only a small portion of patients with tumours smaller than 1 cm with negative axillary SLN and positive IM SLN. Second, the local recurrence rate in the IM region has been found to be low (<1%) amongst patients who had undergone modified radical mastectomy and systemic therapy. Third, resection of IM nodes did not reduce loco-regional recurrence in patients with early-stage breast cancer. Moreover, the removal of IM SLN would be associated with higher morbidity and complications like haemorrhage, pneumothorax, etc. on account of relative lack of familiarity with the technique.

7. Axillary Lymph Node Dissection

   A completion ALND is conventionally performed in all cases where the SLNB report indicates positivity for metastasis. However, according to the 2014 American Society of Clinical Oncology (ASCO) guidelines [39], the recommendations for ALND are as follows:

   (a) Three or more metastatic sentinel lymph nodes on SLNB.
   (b) One or two metastatic sentinel lymph nodes on SLNB but who do not desire whole-breast irradiation.
   (c) Presence of gross extra-nodal extension, regardless of the number.

   A completion ALND is not performed in patients with the following:

   (a) No SN metastasis, including the presence of isolated tumour cells in SLN (s)
   (b) Micro-metastasis
   (c) No occult metastasis and no recommended alteration in subsequent adjuvant therapy [55, 56, 62–64].
   (d) One or two SN metastases in patients receiving whole-breast irradiation as part of breast conservation therapy (according to the ACOSOG Z-0011 & IBCSG 23-01 trials).

   Upcoming Techniques

   Novel tracers that have been investigated for localising SNs include indocyanine green (ICG), superparamagnetic iron oxide (SPIO) and microbubble contrast agents. Although these techniques are being practiced by most centres, these are considered investigational until their reliability in identifying sentinel lymph nodes with a low FNR is well established.

   Indocyanine Green

   ICG is a water-soluble green-coloured near-infrared tracer agent and is radiation-free with high tissue penetration. It provides a novel option to use optimal imaging techniques employing near-infrared fluorescence for transcutaneous identification of sentinel lymph nodes. However, there is a lack of guidelines for a standardised procedure. Still, it usually involves injecting 1–2 ml (1–2.5 mg/ml) of ICG into the breast at the sub-areolar or intradermal site, followed by breast massage for 5 min before operating lights are switched off and real-time images of the lymphatics draining into the axilla are obtained using a laser-assisted imaging device. Factors affecting the IR using this method are advanced age and obesity. In general, ICG is a safe diagnostic agent. Owing to its structure which has both hydrophilic and lipophilic components, it strongly binds to plasma proteins, making it a highly suitable agent for the evaluation of the lymphatic system [65]. It also has a shorter half-life with rapid clearance, allowing multiple intra-operative assessments [66]. A meta-analysis of 12 non-randomised comparative studies revealed that injecting ICG provided equal or better results than radioactive colloid in identifying sentinel lymph nodes [67].

Superparamagnetic Iron Oxide

The magnetic tracer agent, SPIO, is injected into the breast at the sub-areolar or intradermal site on the morning of or just before the surgery. A handheld magnetometer is used for visualisation of SNs. Several trials and meta-analyses show SPIO to be non-inferior to the standard technique [68–81]. Zada et al. conducted a meta-analysis of seven studies in which both SPIO and standard tracers were used in each patient. They reported similar results with both techniques in terms of IRs (97.1 vs 96.8%), total lymph nodes retrieved (1.9 vs 1.8 nodes per patient) and FNRs (8.4 vs 10.9%) and showed a 3.9% mean discordance rate between the two techniques [68]. Amongst various magnetic nanoparticles, the most commonly used are Sienna+, Magtrace and Resovist, with iron concentrations of 28.0, 28.0 and 27.9 mg/ml, respectively [82, 83]. Each lymph node has a maximum capacity to accommodate magnetic particles and varies with the lymph node size [84]. Injecting excessive iron would most likely cause artefacts on breast MRI at the injection site and may pose a challenge in patients requiring post-operative MRI like BRCA carriers or patients with tumours not visible on mammography [85]. Therefore, optimising this technique further to reduce the volume of nanoparticles injected during the procedure is important.

Microbubble contrast

The microbubble contrast agent based on the dispersion employs sulphur hexafluoride gas injected intradermally around the areola. Contrast-enhanced ultrasound is used to visualise and follow breast lymphatics to locate and biopsy sentinel lymph nodes [32]. In a meta-analysis of five studies, this technique was found to identify sentinel lymph nodes in 9.3 to 55.2% of patients with a sensitivity of 61 to 89% and a FNR of 6.6 to 39% [86]. Comparative studies with a standard technique are required to validate this technique.

Take Home

1. Sentinel lymph node biopsy is the standard of care in a node- negative axilla in patients with breast cancer.
2. Axillary lymph node dissection is considered obsolete as a staging procedure in these patients.
3. The dual technique (dye + radioisotope) is the gold standard. All other methods need to be compared with the dual technique of SLNB.
4. With advancements in the form of ICG, SPIO and microbubble contrast, we are evolving to make it less invasive and more accurate with minimum FNRs.
5. With various trials, there is an evolution of thought in omitting ALND even in positive SLNB in favourable scenarios. However, these trials (ACOSOG Z-0011 and IBCSG 23-01 trials) need to be evaluated in developing countries before being extrapolated.

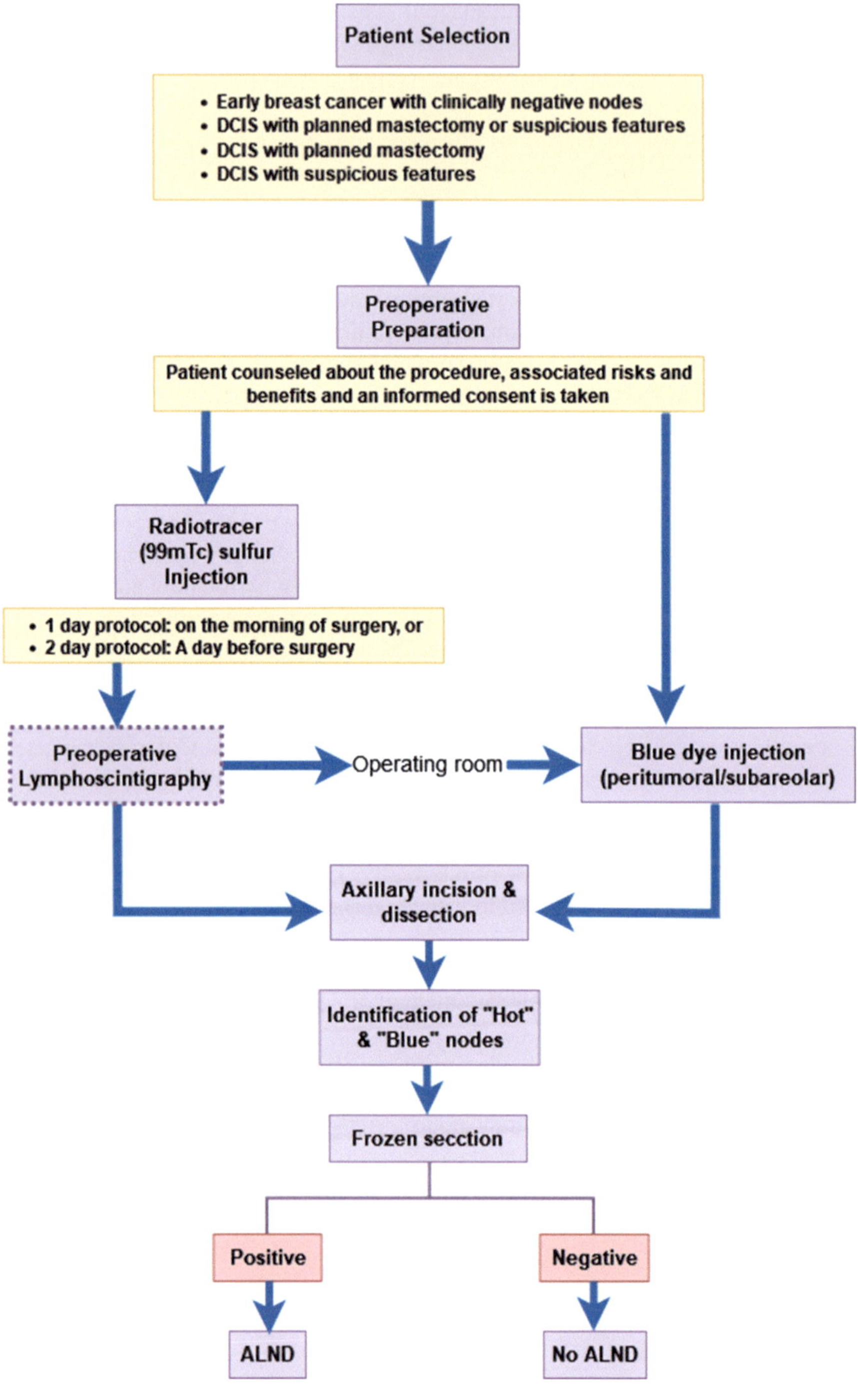
Patient Selection
• Early breast cancer with clinically negative nodes
• DCIS with planned mastectomy or suspicious features
• DCIS with planned mastectomy
• DCIS with suspicious features
Preoperative Preparation
Patient counseled about the procedure, associated risks and benefits and an informed consent is taken
Radiotracer (99mTc) sulfur Injection
• 1 day protocol: on the morning of surgery, or
• 2 day protocol: A day before surgery
Preoperative Lymphoscintigraphy
Operating room
Blue dye injection (peritumoral/subareolar)
Axillary incision & dissection
Identification of "Hot" & "Blue" nodes
Frozen secction
Positive
Negative
ALND
No ALND

References

1. Sacre RA. Clinical evaluation of axillar lymph nodes compared to surgical and pathological findings. Eur J Surg Oncol. 1986;12(2):169–73.
2. Cooper KL, Meng Y, Harnan S, Ward SE, Fitzgerald P, Papaioannou D, et al. Positron emission tomography (PET) and magnetic resonance imaging (MRI) for the assessment of axillary lymph node metastases in early breast cancer: systematic review and economic evaluation. Health Technol Assess. 2011;15(4):iii–v, 1–134. https://doi.org/10.3310/hta15040.
3. Hwang SO, Lee SW, Kim HJ, Kim WW, Park HY, Jung JH. The comparative study of ultrasonography, contrast-enhanced MRI, and (18)F-FDG PET/CT for detecting axillary lymph node metastasis in T1 breast cancer. J Breast Cancer. 2013;16(3):315–21. https://doi.org/10.4048/jbc.2013.16.3.315; Epub 2013 Sep 30.
4. Caudle AS, Cupp JA, Kuerer HM. Management of axillary disease. Surg Oncol Clin N Am. 2014;23(3):473–86. https://doi.org/10.1016/j.soc.2014.03.007; Epub 2014 Apr 13.
5. Krag DN, Weaver DL, Alex JC, Fairbank JT. Surgical resection and radio localization of the sentinel lymph node in breast cancer using a gamma probe. Surg Oncol. 1993;2(6):335–9; discussion 340. https://doi.org/10.1016/0960-7404(93)90064-6.
6. Giuliano AE, Kirgan DM, Guenther JM, Morton DL. Lymphatic mapping and sentinel lymphadenectomy for breast cancer. Ann Surg. 1994;220(3):391–8; discussion 398–401. https://doi.org/10.1097/00000658-199409000-00015.
7. Albertini JJ, Lyman GH, Cox C, Yeatman T, Balducci L, Ku N, et al. Lymphatic mapping and sentinel node biopsy in the patient with breast cancer. JAMA. 1996;276(22):1818–22.
8. Borgstein PJ, Pijpers R, Comans EF, van Diest PJ, Boom RP, Meijer S. Sentinel lymph node biopsy in breast cancer: guidelines and pitfalls of lymphoscintigraphy and gamma probe detection. J Am Coll Surg. 1998;186(3):275–83. https://doi.org/10.1016/s1072-7515(98)00011-8.
9. Radovanovic Z, Golubovic A, Plzak A, Stojiljkovic B, Radovanovic D. Blue dye versus combined blue dye-radioactive tracer technique in detection of sentinel lymph node in breast cancer. Eur J Surg Oncol. 2004;30(9):913–7. https://doi.org/10.1016/j.ejso.2004.08.003.
10. Syme DB, Collins JP, Mann GB. Comparison of blue dye and isotope with blue dye alone in breast sentinel node biopsy. ANZ J Surg. 2005;75(9):817–21. https://doi.org/10.1111/j.1445-2197.2005.03531.x.
11. Hung WK, Chan CM, Ying M, Chong SF, Mak KL, Yip AW. Randomized clinical trial comparing blue dye with combined dye and isotope for sentinel lymph node biopsy in breast cancer. Br J Surg. 2005;92(12):1494–7. https://doi.org/10.1002/bjs.5211.
12. Goyal A, Newcombe RG, Chhabra A, Mansel RE. Factors affecting failed localisation and false-negative rates of sentinel node biopsy in breast cancer–results of the ALMANAC validation phase. Breast Cancer Res Treat. 2006;99(2):203–8. https://doi.org/10.1007/s10549-006-9192-1.
13. Ghiassi S, Sun YS, Kim VB, Scott CM, Nifong LW, Rotondo MF, et al. Methylene blue enhancement of resuscitation after refractory haemorrhagic shock. J Trauma. 2004;57(3):515–21. https://doi.org/10.1097/01.ta.0000136159.22721.3d.
14. Li J, Chen X, Qi M, Li Y. Sentinel lymph node biopsy mapped with methylene blue dye alone in patients with breast cancer: a systematic review and meta-analysis. PLoS One. 2018;13(9):e0204364. https://doi.org/10.1371/journal.pone.0204364.
15. Han C, Yang L, Zuo W. A mini-review on factors and countermeasures associated with false-negative sentinel lymph node biopsies in breast cancer. Chin J Cancer Res. 2016;28(3):370–6. https://doi.org/10.21147/j.issn.1000-9604.2016.03.12.
16. Peek MC, Charalampoudis P, Anninga B, Baker R, Douek M. Blue dye for identification of sentinel nodes in breast cancer and malignant melanoma: a systematic review and meta-analysis. Future Oncol. 2017;13(5):455–67. https://doi.org/10.2217/fon-2016-0255; Epub 2016 Aug 31.
17. Krag DN, Anderson SJ, Julian TB, Brown AM, Harlow SP, Ashikaga T, et al. National Surgical Adjuvant Breast and bowel project. Technical outcomes of sentinel-lymph-node resection

and conventional axillary-lymph-node dissection in patients with clinically node-negative breast cancer: results from the NSABP B-32 randomised phase III trial. Lancet Oncol. 2007;8(10):881–8. https://doi.org/10.1016/S1470-2045(07)70278-4.

18. Raut CP, Hunt KK, Akins JS, Daley MD, Ross MI, Singletary SE, et al. Incidence of anaphylactoid reactions to isosulfan blue dye during breast carcinoma lymphatic mapping in patients treated with preoperative prophylaxis: results of a surgical prospective clinical practice protocol. Cancer. 2005;104(4):692–9. https://doi.org/10.1002/cncr.21226.
19. Wilke LG, McCall LM, Posther KE, Whitworth PW, Reintgen DS, Leitch AM, et al. Surgical complications associated with sentinel lymph node biopsy: results from a prospective international cooperative group trial. Ann Surg Oncol. 2006;13(4):491–500. https://doi.org/10.1245/ASO.2006.05.013; Epub 2006 Mar 2.
20. Perenyei M, Barber ZE, Gibson J, Hemington-Gorse S, Dobbs TD. Anaphylactic reaction rates to blue dyes used for sentinel lymph node mapping: systematic review and meta-analysis. Ann Surg. 2021;273(6):1087–93. https://doi.org/10.1097/SLA.0000000000004061.
21. Brahma B, Putri RI, Karsono R, Andinata B, Gautama W, Sari L, et al. The predictive value of methylene blue dye as a single technique in breast cancer sentinel node biopsy: a study from Dharmais cancer hospital. World J Surg Oncol. 2017;15(1):41. https://doi.org/10.1186/s12957-017-1113-8.
22. Zhang GC, Liao N, Guo ZB, Qian XK, Ren CY, Yao M, et al. Accuracy and axilla sparing potentials of sentinel lymph node biopsy with methylene blue alone performed before versus after neoadjuvant chemotherapy in breast cancer: a single institution experience. Clin Transl Oncol. 2013;15(1):79–84. https://doi.org/10.1007/s12094-012-0885-0; Epub 2012 Aug 28.
23. Bleicher RJ, Kloth DD, Robinson D, Axelrod P. Inflammatory cutaneous adverse effects of methylene blue dye injection for lymphatic mapping/sentinel lymphadenectomy. J Surg Oncol. 2009;99(6):356–60. https://doi.org/10.1002/jso.21240.
24. Teknos D, Ramcharan A, Oluwole SF. Pulmonary edema associated with methylene blue dye administration during sentinel lymph node biopsy. J Natl Med Assoc. 2008;100(12):1483–4. https://doi.org/10.1016/s0027-9684(15)31552-2.
25. Zakaria S, Hoskin TL, Degnim AC. Safety and technical success of methylene blue dye for lymphatic mapping in breast cancer. Am J Surg. 2008;196(2):228–33. https://doi.org/10.1016/j.amjsurg.2007.08.060.
26. Li N, Wang X, Lin B, Zhu H, Liu C, Xu X, et al. Clinical evaluation of 99mTc-rituximab for sentinel lymph node mapping in breast cancer patients. J Nucl Med. 2016;57(8):1214–20. https://doi.org/10.2967/jnumed.115.160572; Epub 2016 Mar 16.
27. İlem-Özdemir D, Yararbas U, Zengel B, Ertan G, Asikoglu M. Preparation of ^{99m}Tc-isosulfan blue for lymph node localization in rats ^{99m}Tc-isosulfan blue for lymph node localization. Appl Radiat Isot. 2016;118:338–42. https://doi.org/10.1016/j.apradiso.2016.10.007; Epub 2016 Oct 11.
28. Nieweg OE, Jansen L, Valdés Olmos RA, Rutgers EJ, Peterse JL, Hoefnagel KA, et al. Lymphatic mapping and sentinel lymph node biopsy in breast cancer. Eur J Nucl Med. 1999;26(4 Suppl):S11–6. https://doi.org/10.1007/s002590050572.
29. Sappey MPC. Injection preparation et conservation des vaisseaux lymphatiques. These pour le doctorat en medecine. No. 241. Paris: Rignoux Imprimeur de la Faculte de Medecine; 1834.
30. Pelosi E, Bellò M, Giors M, Ala A, Giani R, Bussone R, et al. Sentinel lymph node detection in patients with early-stage breast cancer: comparison of periareolar and subdermal/peritumoral injection techniques. J Nucl Med. 2004;45(2):220–5.
31. Giuliano AE, Jones RC, Brennan M, Statman R. Sentinel lymphadenectomy in breast cancer. J Clin Oncol. 1997;15(6):2345–50. https://doi.org/10.1200/JCO.1997.15.6.2345.
32. Cox K, Sever A, Jones S, Weeks J, Mills P, Devalia H, et al. Validation of a technique using microbubbles and contrast enhanced ultrasound (CEUS) to biopsy sentinel lymph nodes (SLN) in pre-operative breast cancer patients with a normal grey-scale axillary ultrasound. Eur J Surg Oncol. 2013;39(7):760–5. https://doi.org/10.1016/j.ejso.2013.03.026; Epub 2013 Apr 28.

33. Kern KA. Concordance and validation study of sentinel lymph node biopsy for breast cancer using subareolar injection of blue dye and technetium 99m sulfur colloid. J Am Coll Surg. 2002;195(4):467–75. https://doi.org/10.1016/s1072-7515(02)01312-1.

34. Veronesi U, Paganelli G, Galimberti V, Viale G, Zurrida S, Bedoni M, et al. Sentinel-node biopsy to avoid axillary dissection in breast cancer with clinically negative lymph-nodes. Lancet. 1997;349(9069):1864–7. https://doi.org/10.1016/S0140-6736(97)01004-0.

35. Rodier JF, Velten M, Wilt M, Martel P, Ferron G, Vaini-Elies V, et al. Prospective multicentric randomized study comparing periareolar and peritumoral injection of radiotracer and blue dye for the detection of sentinel lymph node in breast sparing procedures: FRANSENODE trial. J Clin Oncol. 2007;25(24):3664–9. https://doi.org/10.1200/JCO.2006.08.4228; Epub 2007 May 7.

36. Borgstein PJ, Meijer S, Pijpers RJ, van Diest PJ. Functional lymphatic anatomy for sentinel node biopsy in breast cancer: echoes from the past and the periareolar blue method. Ann Surg. 2000;232(1):81–9. https://doi.org/10.1097/00000658-200007000-00012.

37. Bauer TW, Bedrosian I, Spitz F, et al Subareolar injection simplifies sentinel lymph node mapping for breast cancer [Abstract]. Society of surgical oncology 54th annual cancer symposium; 2001 March 15–18; Washington, DC: Abstract 71.

38. Mudun A, Sanli Y, Ozmen V, Turkmen C, Ozel S, Eroglu A, et al. Comparison of different injection sites of radionuclide for sentinel lymph node detection in breast cancer: single institution experience. Clin Nucl Med. 2008;33(4):262–7. https://doi.org/10.1097/RLU.0b013e3181662fc7.

39. Lyman GH, Giuliano AE, Somerfield MR, Benson AB 3rd, Bodurka DC, Burstein HJ, et al. American Society of Clinical Oncology. American Society of Clinical Oncology guideline recommendations for sentinel lymph node biopsy in early-stage breast cancer. J Clin Oncol. 2005;23(30):7703–20. https://doi.org/10.1200/JCO.2005.08.001; Epub 2005 Sep 12.

40. Shimazu K, Tamaki Y, Taguchi T, Motomura K, Inaji H, Koyama H, et al. Lymphoscintigraphic visualization of internal mammary nodes with subtumoral injection of radiocolloid in patients with breast cancer. Ann Surg. 2003;237(3):390–8. https://doi.org/10.1097/01.SLA.0000055226.89022.90.

41. Tanis PJ, Deurloo EE, Valdés Olmos RA, Rutgers EJ, Nieweg OE, Besnard AP, et al. Single intralesional tracer dose for radio-guided excision of clinically occult breast cancer and sentinel node. Ann Surg Oncol. 2001;8(10):850–5. https://doi.org/10.1007/s10434-001-0850-6.

42. Doting MH, Jansen L, Nieweg OE, Piers DA, Tiebosch AT, Koops HS, et al. Lymphatic mapping with intralesional tracer administration in breast carcinoma patients. Cancer. 2000;88(11):2546–52.

43. van der Ploeg IM, Tanis PJ, Valdés Olmos RA, Kroon BB, Rutgers EJ, Nieweg OE. Breast cancer patients with extra-axillary sentinel nodes only may be spared axillary lymph node dissection. Ann Surg Oncol. 2008;15(11):3239–43. https://doi.org/10.1245/s10434-008-0120-y; Epub 2008 Sep 5.

44. Krag D, Weaver D, Ashikaga T, Moffat F, Klimberg VS, Shriver C, et al. The sentinel node in breast cancer--a multicenter validation study. N Engl J Med. 1998;339(14):941–6. https://doi.org/10.1056/NEJM199810013391401.

45. Veronesi U, Paganelli G, Viale G, Galimberti V, Luini A, Zurrida S, et al. Sentinel lymph node biopsy and axillary dissection in breast cancer: results in a large series. J Natl Cancer Inst. 1999;91(4):368–73. https://doi.org/10.1093/jnci/91.4.368.

46. Miner TJ, Shriver CD, Flicek PR, Miner FC, Jaques DP, Maniscalco-Theberge ME, et al. Guidelines for the safe use of radioactive materials during localization and resection of the sentinel lymph node. Ann Surg Oncol. 1999;6(1):75–82. https://doi.org/10.1007/s10434-999-0075-7.

47. Cox CE, Pendas S, Cox JM, Joseph E, Shons AR, Yeatman T, et al. Guidelines for sentinel node biopsy and lymphatic mapping of patients with breast cancer. Ann Surg. 1998;227(5):645–51; discussion 651–3. https://doi.org/10.1097/00000658-199805000-00005.

48. McMasters KM, Wong SL, Tuttle TM, Carlson DJ, Brown CM, Dirk Noyes R, et al. Preoperative lymphoscintigraphy for breast cancer does not improve the ability to

identify axillary sentinel lymph nodes. Ann Surg. 2000;231(5):724–31. https://doi.org/10.1097/00000658-200005000-00013.
49. Burak WE Jr, Walker MJ, Yee LD, Kim JA, Saha S, Hinkle G, et al. Routine preoperative lymphoscintigraphy is not necessary prior to sentinel node biopsy for breast cancer. Am J Surg. 1999;177(6):445–9. https://doi.org/10.1016/s0002-9610(99)00088-4.
50. Wang L, Yu JM, Wang YS, Zuo WS, Gao Y, Fan J, Li JY, Hu XD, Chen ML, Yang GR, Zhou ZB, Liu YS, Li YQ, Liu YB, Zhao T, Chen P. Preoperative lymphoscintigraphy predicts the successful identification but is not necessary in sentinel lymph nodes biopsy in breast cancer. Ann Surg Oncol. 2007;14(8):2215–20. https://doi.org/10.1245/s10434-007-9418-4; Epub 2007 May 24.
51. Martin RC 2nd, Edwards MJ, Wong SL, Tuttle TM, Carlson DJ, Brown CM, et al. Practical guidelines for optimal gamma probe detection of sentinel lymph nodes in breast cancer: results of a multi-institutional study. For the University of Louisville Breast Cancer Study Group. Surgery. 2000;128(2):139–44. https://doi.org/10.1067/msy.2000.108064.
52. Chung A, Yu J, Stempel M, Patil S, Cody H, Montgomery L. Is the "10% rule" equally valid for all subsets of sentinel-node-positive breast cancer patients? Ann Surg Oncol. 2008;15(10):2728–33. https://doi.org/10.1245/s10434-008-0050-8; Epub 2008 Aug 8.
53. American Joint Committee on Cancer. In: Edge SB, editor. Cancer staging manual. 7th ed. New York: Springer; 2010. p. 347.
54. Giuliano AE, Connolly JL, Edge SB, Mittendorf EA, Rugo HS, Solin LJ, et al. Breast cancer-major changes in the American Joint Committee on Cancer eighth edition cancer staging manual. CA Cancer J Clin. 2017;67(4):290–303. https://doi.org/10.3322/caac.21393; Epub 2017 Mar 14. Erratum in: CA Cancer J Clin. 2017 Jul 8;67(4):345.
55. Weaver DL, Ashikaga T, Krag DN, Skelly JM, Anderson SJ, Harlow SP, et al. Effect of occult metastases on survival in node-negative breast cancer. N Engl J Med. 2011;364(5):412–21. https://doi.org/10.1056/NEJMoa1008108; Epub 2011 Jan 19.
56. Giuliano AE, Hawes D, Ballman KV, Whitworth PW, Blumencranz PW, Reintgen DS, et al. Association of occult metastases in sentinel lymph nodes and bone marrow with survival among women with early-stage invasive breast cancer. JAMA. 2011;306(4):385–93. https://doi.org/10.1001/jama.2011.1034.
57. Choi AH, Surrusco M, Rodriguez S, Bahjri K, Solomon N, Garberoglio C, et al. Extranodal extension on sentinel lymph node dissection: why should we treat it differently? Am Surg. 2014;80(10):932–5.
58. Changsri C, Prakash S, Sandweiss L, Bose S. Prediction of additional axillary metastasis of breast cancer following sentinel lymph node surgery. Breast J. 2004;10(5):392–7. https://doi.org/10.1111/j.1075-122X.2004.21446.x.
59. Abdessalam SF, Zervos EE, Prasad M, Farrar WB, Yee LD, Walker MJ, et al. Predictors of positive axillary lymph nodes after sentinel lymph node biopsy in breast cancer. Am J Surg. 2001;182(4):316–20. https://doi.org/10.1016/s0002-9610(01)00719-x.
60. McMasters KM, Tuttle TM, Carlson DJ, Brown CM, Noyes RD, Glaser RL, et al. Sentinel lymph node biopsy for breast cancer: a suitable alternative to routine axillary dissection in multi-institutional practice when optimal technique is used. J Clin Oncol. 2000;18(13):2560–6. https://doi.org/10.1200/JCO.2000.18.13.2560.
61. Klauber-DeMore N, Bevilacqua JL, Van Zee KJ, Borgen P, Cody HS 3rd. Comprehensive review of the management of internal mammary lymph node metastases in breast cancer. J Am Coll Surg. 2001;193(5):547–55. https://doi.org/10.1016/s1072-7515(01)01040-7.
62. Reed J, Rosman M, Verbanac KM, Mannie A, Cheng Z, Tafra L. Prognostic implications of isolated tumor cells and micrometastases in sentinel nodes of patients with invasive breast cancer: 10-year analysis of patients enrolled in the prospective East Carolina University/Anne Arundel medical center sentinel node multicenter study. J Am Coll Surg. 2009;208(3):333–40. https://doi.org/10.1016/j.jamcollsurg.2008.10.036; Epub 2008 Dec 25.
63. Chagpar A, Middleton LP, Sahin AA, Meric-Bernstam F, Kuerer HM, Feig BW, et al. Clinical outcome of patients with lymph node-negative breast carcinoma who have sentinel lymph

node micrometastases detected by immunohistochemistry. Cancer. 2005;103(8):1581–6. https://doi.org/10.1002/cncr.20934.

64. Pugliese MS, Beatty JD, Tickman RJ, Allison KH, Atwood MK, Szymonifka J, et al. Impact and outcomes of routine microstaging of sentinel lymph nodes in breast cancer: significance of the pN0(i+) and pN1mi categories. Ann Surg Oncol. 2009;16(1):113–20. https://doi.org/10.1245/s10434-008-0121-x; Epub 2008 Oct 23.
65. Kogure K, David NJ, Yamanouchi U, Choromokos E. Infrared absorption angiography of the fundus circulation. Arch Ophthalmol. 1970;83(2):209–14. https://doi.org/10.1001/archopht.1970.00990030211015.
66. Elite system Spy. Elite system SPY: kit instructions for use. Branchburg, NJ: LifeCell corp; 2011.
67. Sugie T, Ikeda T, Kawaguchi A, Shimizu A, Toi M. Sentinel lymph node biopsy using indocyanine green fluorescence in early-stage breast cancer: a meta-analysis. Int J Clin Oncol. 2017;22(1):11–7. https://doi.org/10.1007/s10147-016-1064-z; Epub 2016 Nov 19.
68. Zada A, Peek MC, Ahmed M, Anninga B, Baker R, Kusakabe M, et al. Meta-analysis of sentinel lymph node biopsy in breast cancer using the magnetic technique. Br J Surg. 2016;103(11):1409–19. https://doi.org/10.1002/bjs.10283; Epub 2016 Sep 9.
69. Douek M, Klaase J, Monypenny I, Kothari A, Zechmeister K, Brown D, et al. Sentinel node biopsy using a magnetic tracer versus standard technique: the SentiMAG multicentre trial. Ann Surg Oncol. 2014;21(4):1237–45. https://doi.org/10.1245/s10434-013-3379-6; Epub 2013 Dec 10.
70. Thill M, Kurylcio A, Welter R, van Haasteren V, Grosse B, Berclaz G, et al. The central-European SentiMag study: sentinel lymph node biopsy with superparamagnetic iron oxide (SPIO) vs. radioisotope. Breast. 2014;23(2):175–9. https://doi.org/10.1016/j.breast.2014.01.004; Epub 2014 Jan 29.
71. Shiozawa M, Lefor AT, Hozumi Y, Kurihara K, Sata N, Yasuda Y, et al. Sentinel lymph node biopsy in patients with breast cancer using superparamagnetic iron oxide and a magnetometer. Breast Cancer. 2013;20(3):223–9. https://doi.org/10.1007/s12282-011-0327-9; Epub 2012 Jan 13.
72. Rubio IT, Diaz-Botero S, Esgueva A, Rodriguez R, Cortadellas T, Cordoba O, Espinosa-Bravo M. The superparamagnetic iron oxide is equivalent to the Tc99 radiotracer method for identifying the sentinel lymph node in breast cancer. Eur J Surg Oncol. 2015;41(1):46–51. https://doi.org/10.1016/j.ejso.2014.11.006; Epub 2014 Nov 15.
73. Piñero-Madrona A, Torró-Richart JA, de León-Carrillo JM, de Castro-Parga G, Navarro-Cecilia J, Domínguez-Cunchillos F, et al. Grupo de Estudios Senológicos de la Sociedad Española de Patologia Mamaria (SESPM). Superparamagnetic iron oxide as a tracer for sentinel node biopsy in breast cancer: A comparative non-inferiority study. Eur J Surg Oncol. 2015;41(8):991–7. https://doi.org/10.1016/j.ejso.2015.04.017; Epub 2015 May 12.
74. Houpeau JL, Chauvet MP, Guillemin F, Bendavid-Athias C, Charitansky H, Kramar A, et al. Sentinel lymph node identification using superparamagnetic iron oxide particles versus radioisotope: the French Sentimag feasibility trial. J Surg Oncol. 2016;113(5):501–7. https://doi.org/10.1002/jso.24164; Epub 2016 Jan 12.
75. Ghilli M, Carretta E, Di Filippo F, Battaglia C, Fustaino L, Galanou I, et al. The superparamagnetic iron oxide tracer: a valid alternative in sentinel node biopsy for breast cancer treatment. Eur J Cancer Care (Engl). 2017;26(4) https://doi.org/10.1111/ecc.12385; Epub 2015 Sep 14.
76. Ahmed M, Purushotham AD, Douek M. Novel techniques for sentinel lymph node biopsy in breast cancer: a systematic review. Lancet Oncol. 2014;15(8):e351–62. https://doi.org/10.1016/S1470-2045(13)70590-4.
77. Karakatsanis A, Christiansen PM, Fischer L, Hedin C, Pistioli L, Sund M, et al. The Nordic SentiMag trial: a comparison of super paramagnetic iron oxide (SPIO) nanoparticles versus Tc(99) and patent blue in the detection of sentinel node (SN) in patients with breast cancer and a meta-analysis of earlier studies. Breast Cancer Res Treat. 2016;157(2):281–94. https://doi.org/10.1007/s10549-016-3809-9; Epub 2016 Apr 27.

78. Teshome M, Wei C, Hunt KK, Thompson A, Rodriguez K, Mittendorf EA. Use of a magnetic tracer for sentinel lymph node detection in early-stage breast cancer patients: a meta-analysis. Ann Surg Oncol. 2016;23(5):1508–14. https://doi.org/10.1245/s10434-016-5135-1; Epub 2016 Feb 18.
79. Alvarado MD, Mittendorf EA, Teshome M, Thompson AM, Bold RJ, Gittleman MA, et al. A non-inferiority trial comparing superparamagnetic iron oxide versus technetium-99m and blue dye in the detection of axillary sentinel nodes in patients with early-stage breast cancer. Ann Surg Oncol. 2019;26(11):3510–6. https://doi.org/10.1245/s10434-019-07577-4; Epub 2019 Jul 11. Erratum in: Ann Surg Oncol. 2020 Dec;27(Suppl 3):979.
80. Hersi AF, Pistiolis L, Dussan Luberth C, Vikhe-Patil E, Nilsson F, Mohammed I, et al. Optimizing dose and timing in magnetic tracer techniques for sentinel lymph node detection in early breast cancers: the prospective multicenter SentiDose trial. Cancers (Basel). 2021;13(4):693. https://doi.org/10.3390/cancers13040693.
81. Taruno K, Kurita T, Kuwahata A, Yanagihara K, Enokido K, Katayose Y, et al. Multicenter clinical trial on sentinel lymph node biopsy using superparamagnetic iron oxide nanoparticles and a novel handheld magnetic probe. J Surg Oncol. 2019;120(8):1391–6. https://doi.org/10.1002/jso.25747; Epub 2019 Oct 30.
82. Pouw JJ, Ahmed M, Anninga B, Schuurman K, Pinder SE, Van Hemelrijck M, et al. Comparison of three magnetic nanoparticle tracers for sentinel lymph node biopsy in an in vivo porcine model. Int J Nanomedicine. 2015;10:1235–43. https://doi.org/10.2147/IJN.S76962.
83. Rubio IT, Rodriguez-Revuelto R, Espinosa-Bravo M, Siso C, Rivero J, Esgueva A. A randomized study comparing different doses of superparamagnetic iron oxide tracer for sentinel lymph node biopsy in breast cancer: the SUNRISE study. Eur J Surg Oncol. 2020;46(12):2195–201. https://doi.org/10.1016/j.ejso.2020.06.018; Epub 2020 Jun 18.
84. Peek MCL, Saeki K, Ohashi K, Chikaki S, Baker R, Nakagawa T, et al. Optimization of SPIO injection for sentinel lymph node dissection in a rat model. Cancers (Basel). 2021;13(19):5031. https://doi.org/10.3390/cancers13195031.
85. Huizing E, Anninga B, Young P, Monypenny I, Hall-Craggs M, Douek M. Analysis of void artefacts in post-operative breast MRI due to residual SPIO after magnetic SLNB in SentiMAG trial participants. Eur J Surg Oncol. 2015;41:S18. https://doi.org/10.1016/j.ejso.2015.03.005.
86. Gkegkes ID, Iavazzo C. Contrast enhanced ultrasound (CEU) using microbubbles for sentinel lymph node biopsy in breast cancer: a systematic review. Acta Chir Belg. 2015;115(3):212–8. https://doi.org/10.1080/00015458.2015.11681099.

Complications of SLNB in Breast Cancer

6

Elina Shaari and Hisham Hamed

6.1 Introduction

Breast cancer is a historic disease. The first written documentation describing breast cancer was in Edwin Smith Papyrus in 3000 BC [1]. Since then, there have been several theories attempting to explain possible underlying causes of breast cancer; none of them were scientifically based. It was not until much later that the nature of breast cancer began to unravel [2].

A fundamental aspect of understanding cancer is to understand its behaviour and importantly the mode of its spread. It was not until the mid-eighteenth century when Le Dran proposed the spread of breast cancer via lymphatic channels [2].

Regional lymph nodes, particularly axillary nodal status, have been established over time as the most important prognostic factor [3] in the history of breast cancer. Consequently, it has become the focus of attention, and extensive research to ascertain the most appropriate and effective way of managing this anatomical region has been subject of extensive research.

Breast cancer is the most common among female cancers. It affects over 1.3 million women worldwide. Advances in the treatment of breast cancer have significantly improved survival and have left a substantial and increasing number of women alive with history of the disease. Consequently, the impact of treatment, albeit curative, on quality of life has become a fundamental part of treatment strategies, and careful assessment of outcome of treatment modality, ascertaining the balance between oncological benefits, drawbacks and complications, has become a central part of modern and holistic approach to treatment of breast cancer.

E. Shaari · H. Hamed (✉)
Department of Breast Surgery, Guy's & St. Thomas' NHS Foundation Trust, London, UK

Chintamani (ed.), *Sentinel Node Biopsy in Breast Cancer*,
https://doi.org/10.1007/978-81-322-3994-9_6

6.2 Surgical Management of the Axilla

Axillary lymph node involvement had been considered not only as an important prognostic indicator but also an important component of local control of breast cancer. There has been no combination of predictors of axillary node status to replace information obtained by surgery and histological examination.

In the mid-sixteenth century, Marcus Aurelius Severino was the first to report removal of enlarged axillary nodes in breast cancer patients.

Henry Le Dran reasoned that if axillary node involvement was indicative of poor prognosis at the early stage of breast cancer, eliminating it by surgical excision before further spread should improve the outcome. Jean Louis Petit (1674–1750) was first to propose en bloc resection of the breast and palpable axillary lymph nodes. However, it was not until the end of the nineteenth century that radical mastectomy became the standard of care advocated and popularised by William Halsted [4].

The increase in women's awareness, introduction of breast screening and technological advances have led to earlier detection of breast cancer with consequently lower incidences of axillary nodal involvement.

Therefore, routine radical resection of axillary nodes, with no clinical evidence of involvement, not only became oncologically non-beneficial but instead likely detrimental to patients' well-being and quality of life.

It became crucial therefore to establish a procedure that allows accurate staging of the axilla to aid in appropriate management without unacceptable co-morbidity. Krag and Giuliano reported the sentinel lymph node biopsy (SLNB) technique for the axilla, in the management of breast cancer, in 1993 and 1994 [5, 6].

SLNB, as an alternative to axillary lymph node dissection (ALND), discussed in other chapters, has been established as the standard of care in patients with invasive breast cancer with no clinical evidence of axillary lymph node metastases since the early 2000s [7].

ALND has been associated with significant and frequent co-morbidity, namely, lymphoedema, seroma formation, compromised arm functions and sensory changes [8].

SLNB itself is not without drawbacks and complications. However, these complications are reported much less frequently compared with ALND. Giuliano et al. reported an overall complication rate of only 3% following SLNB versus 35% in SLNB/ALND [9].

6.3 Complications

This chapter focuses on the many complications associated with any axillary surgery, including SLNB. However, other rare complications have also been encountered.

6.3.1 Lymphoedema

This is the most significant sequelae of axillary surgery, including that following SLNB.

Lymphatic channels are disrupted during the SLNB procedure. This leads to the build-up of interstitial lymph fluid, which in turn causes swelling, secondary to lymphoedema and fibroadipose proliferative activity [10]. These changes cause discomfort, and the affected area may be susceptible to infection/cellulitis.

Lymphoedema progresses through four stages. Stage 0 indicates a normal extremity clinically but with abnormal lymph transport (illustrated by lymphoscintigraphy). Stage 1 is early oedema, which improves with limb elevation. Stage 2 represents pitting oedema that does not resolve with elevation. Stage 3 describes fibroadipose deposition and skin changes [11].

The severity of lymphoedema is categorised as mild (<20% increase in extremity volume), moderate (20–40%) or severe (>40%) [12].

The clinical extent of lymphoedema varies from swelling of fingers only, wrist swelling, forearm swelling or lymphoedema affecting the whole arm. Symptomatic reporting of arm swelling was 3% following SLNB to 27% after ALND. Reported arm swelling did not coincide with measurable lymphoedema. Measurable lymphoedema coincided more with reported symptomatic swelling of the arm. Following SLNB, lymphoedema was reported less frequently (5%) than following SLNB/ALND (16%). In general, only 41% of patients who reported arm swelling had measurable lymphoedema, whereas measurable lymphoedema was found only in 5% of asymptomatic patients [13]. This discordance between symptoms and measurable lymphoedema is of importance when reporting the incidence of lymphoedema and should be clearly stated.

There are several methods for measuring and assessing the extent of lymphoedema. Limb volume measurements can be made using a tape measure or porometer or by water displacement. Tape measurements are the least accurate method to determine volume; it is also difficult to use the exact reference points for future assessments.

There is a significant variation in the risk of lymphoedema reported, ranging from 7 to 77% after ALND and 0 to 13% after SLNB [13]. After one of the earliest SLNB trials, arm lymphoedema following SLNB was reported to occur in approximate 5% of cases (ALMANAC trial) [14].

Lymphoedema is a chronic condition and is associated with lifetime risk. After 3 years, 25% of cases develop lymphoedema.

Early arm exercise encourages collateral channels to open up and could contribute to reduced risk and extent of lymphoedema. Therefore it is important to detect lymphoedema at an early stage for physiotherapy to have a beneficial outcome. Lymphoedema rate increases with the number of LNs removed, which is a factor that contributes to lower risk of lymphoedema after SLNB compared with ALND.

Chronic lymphoedema can also be complicated by a serious consequence, such as lymphangiosarcoma or the Stewart–Treves syndrome (STS). It is a very rare aggressive malignancy with grave prognosis, which was reported in 1948 by Stewart and Treves in a series of 6 cases with chronic lymphoedema following radical mastectomy. It represents only less than 1% of all sarcomas. The risk emerges after 8–24 years. This condition is fatal and attempted surgery is radical amounting to quadrantectomy. Histological diagnosis is essential to differentiate from other malignancies. Surgical treatment is often radical involving amputation or disarticulation of the shoulder. However, unfortunately, the extent of surgery does not affect the poor prognosis [15, 16].

6.3.2 Seroma Formation

Seroma is a consequence of any surgery and not strictly an exclusive complication of ALND or SLNB procedure. It is the result of reactionary interstitial fluid build-up in the potential space left by excised tissue. This is a natural reaction of the body to injury. The body usually absorbs a small seroma. However, a large build-up causing tense swelling and pain will require percutaneous drainage, preferably under radiological guidance to avoid injury to other axillary structures/vessels.

6.3.3 Arm/Shoulder Mobility

Axillary surgery is associated with other extremity's comorbidity, which is related to the extent of surgery. One of the earliest SLNB trials [14] has shown a significantly better functionality of the arm after SLNB compared with ALND. Purushotham et al. had shown that shoulder mobility was less impaired after SLNB compared with ALND [8]. However, the difference was only significant in the early post-operative period and diminished over subsequent 3 months of post-operative period.

6.3.4 Nerve Injury and Sensory Changes

Numbness and paraesthesia of the upper arm and axillary region were reported in 70–80% of cases following ALND [17]. Numbness remains the most prevalent sensory change, observed in 55% versus 22% in ALND and SLNB, respectively [13].

The cutaneous branches of the sensory nerves are likely to be cut when skin incision is made or dissection is carried out. ICBNs are the most common sensory nerves encountered in the axilla. They usually originate from the lateral cutaneous branch of the second and forth intercostal nerves. Henry and Kumar described that these nerves traverse the axilla to terminally supply the region of the medial arm [18, 19]. They function to provide sensory innervation to the axilla, lateral chest and medial upper arm [20, 21]. The proximity and course of the ICBNs in relation to axillary contents and lymph nodes pose a danger of iatrogenic injury during axillary surgery, and such injury has been associated with post-operative sensory loss and neuropathic pain [20, 22].

A meta-analysis by Henry et al. [18] reported that a total of 16 studies (1567 axillae) reported data indicating that the ICBNs were present in 98.4% of cases. It most often (90.6%) originated from fibres at the T2 spinal level and commonly coursed in two branching patterns: as a single trunk in 47.0% of cases and as a bifurcating pattern in 42.2%. In the latter cases, the bifurcation was usually unequal (63.4%). Such an anatomical variation does explain the varying degrees of post-operative sensory changes.

To minimise such a distressing complication, surgeons need to exercise caution to preserve the ICBNs whenever possible, without compromising oncological safety. Ultimately careful dissection and knowledge of ICBN anatomy could lead to reduction in this post-operative complication and improve patient's quality of life [18].

In reviewing the SLNB techniques, it was suggested that accurate localisation of the site of SLN with the aid of lymphoscintigraphy and skin marking reduced the risk of damaging ICBNs. There is limited benefit of lymphoscintigraphy with increasing surgical dexterity. With the current worldwide practice of dual-technique method for SLNB, employing a handheld gamma probe as a radioisotope tracer and tracking a blue dye, combined with careful dissection, preserving ICBNs is often successful.

In view of the limited extent of surgery, reduced frequency of sensory changes can be achieved with SLNB [23].

6.3.5 Axillary Web Syndrome (AWS)

AWS refers to fibrotic band, cord, secondary to sclerosed veins and lymphatics with surrounding fibrosis. This is seen following axillary surgery particularly ALND. It is also seen following SLNB but much less frequently. AWS is reported in up to 72% and 20% following ALND and SLNB, respectively. It is also reported in cases with extensive axillary nodal involvement. AWS sometime forms subcutaneous nodules and should be distinguished from breast cancer recurrence [24]. Koehler et al. reported an AWS prevalence of 50% at 18 months [25], and Baggi et al. found a 51% incidence in 8 weeks following surgery [26].

The condition is self-limiting, though physiotherapy and manual lymphatic drainage could accelerate its resolution [27]. AWS is observed in the early post-operative period and significantly decreased incidence after 3 months with no cases reported after 1 year.

6.3.6 Anaphylactic Reaction to Blue Dye

The SLN can be located by intra-parenchymal or subcutaneous injection of blue dye, either alone or in combination with a radiotracer. Isosulfan blue (IB) is a patent dye, which is absorbed by the lymphoid tissue. The blue dye is used for lymphatic mapping and identification of sentinel lymph nodes.

In a large study involving 1456 patients with breast cancer who underwent SLNB using both blue dye and radionucleotide, a range of adverse reactions were reported in 0.06–2.7% of cases with a mean risk of 0.71%. Symptoms ranged from mild urticaria and erythema to severe, pulmonary oedema, hypotension and cerebrovascular collapse. A total of 12 patients (0.8%) in this study had severe anaphylactic reactions. All 12 patients experienced cardiovascular collapse and skin reactions. These patients required admission to a high dependency unit for post-operative management. There were no deaths or permanent disability reported.

The symptoms tend to manifest within 15–30 min from the time of injection. Early detection and prompt action are crucial to avoid any serious consequences [28].

Montogomery et al. classified reaction to blue dye into three grades: G1 as mild urticaria, G2 with mild hypotension requiring no treatment and G3 with severe hypotension requiring vasopressors [29].

Though reaction to blue dye is a rare event, blue dye should not be used in pregnant women or those with known reaction to the dye. Isosulfan blue reaction was reported in 1.4% of cases when the dye was used [26].

In the UK, the Patent V blue dye (an isomer of isosulphan) is used in combination with the radioactive (TcM99m) labelled nano-colloid. This dual technique has led to the identification of SLN in 99% of patients.

Patent V blue is a colouring used in textiles and food (E131). NEW START and ALMANAC, the largest UK SLNB datasets, demonstrated a 1% allergy rate in nearly 6000 procedures [30]. No mortality has been reported. The majority of these reactions were grade 1, but non-fatal cardio-respiratory arrest has been reported elsewhere [31].

Another blue dye used for SLNB is methylene blue. It is used less commonly because of concerns regarding lymphatic uptake and fat necrosis at the injection site but appears to have less reported allergy reactions.

Every effort must be made to minimise risk to the patient. With around 55,000 new breast cancer cases diagnosed annually in the UK, and a significant proportion likely to undergo SLNB (up to 70%), a 1% reaction rate would equate to potentially 400 adverse events annually. The patient must be counselled regarding blue dye use and its reaction rate and documented on the consent form. For those with serious history of allergy or known allergy to food colourings, a pre-operative skin patch testing can be performed, and if positive, blue dye should be avoided, at the risk of lower detection rates. In these cases, the patient should be counselled for axillary sampling.

6.3.7 Wound Infection: SSI

This is another common consequence of any surgery, not exclusive to SLNB procedures. Breast surgery is categorised as "clean" procedure and carries the lowest risk (2–4%) for surgical site infection (SSI) [32].

Nevertheless, post-chemotherapy, obesity, diabetes, smoking or use of immunosuppressants can lead to an increased risk of wound infection, and intra-operative prophylactic antibiotics is recommended in these cases.

6.4 Conclusion

Advances in breast cancer management and treatment have been associated with significant improvement in survival. Therefore, the quality of life of breast cancer survivors has become an essential aspect of care for these patients.

Radical surgery has been associated with significant chest wall and arm morbidity. The advent of less extensive surgery with the use of breast-conserving surgery, onco-plastic approach and advent of lesser extensive axillary surgery in the form of SLNB has significantly improved patients' quality of life [33].

Moreover, SLNB results in substantially less post-operative morbidity following axillary surgery [34], including wound infection, seroma formation, damage to sensory and motor nerves, pain, loss of arm strength, impaired range of shoulder movements [35] and lymphoedema, which is of particular concern for women undergoing axillary surgery.

It is therefore fundamental in the modern era of cancer therapy that patients' quality of life is prioritized when planning patients' treatment, without of course compromising the oncological aspects.

References

1. Bland KI, Copeland III EM, Klimberg SV. History of the therapy of breast cancer. The Breast (Fifth Edition) 2018. Pages 1–19. e3.
2. https://www.news-medical.net/health/History-of-Breast-Cancer.aspx.
3. Carter CL, Allen C, Henson DE. Relation of tumor size, lymph node status, and survival in 24,740 breast cancer cases. Cancer. 1989;63(1):181–7.
4. Sakorafas GH, Safioleas M. Breast cancer surgery: an historical narrative. Part II. 18th and 19th centuries.
5. Krag DN, Weaver DL, Alex JC, Fairbank JT. Surgical resection and radiolocalization of the sentinel lymph node in breast cancer using a gamma probe. Surg Oncol. 1993;2:335–9.
6. Giuliano AE, Kirgan DM, Guenther JM, Morton DL. Lymphatic mapping and sentinel lymphadenectomy for breast cancer. Ann Surg. 1994;220(3):391.
7. Lyman GH, Giuliano AE, Somerfield MR, et al. American Society of Clinical Oncology guideline recommendations for sentinel lymph node biopsy in early-stage Breast cancer. J Clin Oncol. 2005;23(7):703–20.
8. Purushotham AD, Upponi S, Klevesath MB, Bobrow L, Millar K, Myles JP, Duffy SW. Morbidity after sentinel lymph node biopsy in primary Breast cancer: results from a randomized controlled trial. J Clin Oncol. 2005;23:4312–21.
9. Giuliano AE, Haigh PI, Brennan MB, et al. Prospective observational study of sentinel lymphadenectomy without further axillary dissection in patients with sentinel node-negative breast cancer. J Clin Oncol. 2000;18:2553–9.
10. Brorson H, Ohlin K, Olsson G, Karlsson MK. Breast cancer-related chronic arm lymphedema is associated with excess adipose and muscle tissue. Lymphat Res Biol. 2009;7(1):3–10.

11. Greene A, Goss J. Diagnosis and staging of lymphedema. Semin Plast Surg. 2018;32(1):12–6.
12. The diagnosis and treatment of peripheral lymphedema: 2020 Consensus Document of the International Society of Lymphology.
13. McLaughlin SA, Wright MJ, Morris KT, Sampson MR, Brockway JP, Hurley KE, Riedel ER, Van Zee KJ. Prevalence of lymphedema in women with Breast cancer 5 years after sentinel lymph node biopsy or axillary dissection: patient perceptions and precautionary behaviors. J Clin Oncol. 2008;26:5220–6.
14. Mansel R, et al. Randomised multicentre trial of sentinel node biopsy versus standard axillary treatment in operable Breast cancer: the ALMANAC trial. J Natl Cancer Inst. 2006;98:599–609.
15. Stewart FW. Lymphangiosarcoma in postmastectomy lymphedema; a report of six cases in *Elephantiasis chirurgica*. Cancer. 1948;1:64–81.
16. Mesli SN, Ghouali AK, Benamara F, Taleb FA, Tahraoui H, Abi-Ayad C. Stewart-Treves syndrome involving chronic lymphedema after mastectomy of breast cancer. Case Rep Surg. 2017;2017:4056459.
17. Ivens D, Hoe AL, Podd TJ, et al. Assessment of morbidity from complete axillary dissection. Br J Cancer. 1992;66:136–8.
18. Henry BM, Graves MJ, Pękala JR, Sanna B, Hsieh WC, Tubbs RS, Walocha JA, Tomaszewski KA. Origin, branching, and communications of the intercostobrachial nerve: a meta-analysis with implications for mastectomy and axillary lymph node dissection in breast cancer. Cureus. 2017;9(3):e1101.
19. Kumar P, Meena RN, Sheikh BH, Belliappa V, Pais AV. Intercostobrachial nerve - anatomical considerations and its importance in carcinoma breast of female patients. Ann Surg Perioper Care. 2016;1(2):1013.
20. Mewa Kinoo S, Singh B. Complex regional pain syndrome of the breast and chest wall. Breast J. 2016;22(3):366–8.
21. Soares EW. Anatomical variations of the axilla. Springerplus. 2014;3:306.
22. Zhu JJ, Liu XF, Zhang PL, Yang JZ, Wang J, Qin Y, Zhang GL, Ren DQ, Cui CL, Guo XG. Anatomical information for intercostobrachial nerve preservation in axillary lymph node dissection for breast cancer. Genet Mol Res. 2014;13(4):9315–23.
23. Kim SC, Kim DW, Moadel RM, Kim CK, Chatterjee S, Shafir MK, Travis A, Machac J, Krynyckyi BR. Using the intraoperative handheld probe without lymphoscintigraphy or using only dye correlates with higher sensory morbidity following sentinel lymph node biopsy in breast cancer: a review of the literature. World J Surg Oncol. 2005;3:64.
24. Dinas K, Kalder M, Zepiridis L, Mavromatidis G, Pratilas G. Axillary web syndrome: incidence, pathogenesis, and management. Curr Probl Cancer. 2019;43:100470.
25. Koehler LA, Hunter DW, Blaes AH, Haddad TC. Function, shoulder motion, pain, and lymphedema in breast cancer with and without axillary web syndrome: an 18-month follow-up. Phys Ther. 2018;98(6):518–27.
26. Baggi F, Nevola Teixeira LF, Gandini S, et al. Axillary web syndrome assessment using a self-assessment questionnaire: a prospective cohort study. Support Care Cancer. 2018;26(8):2801–7.
27. Lauridsen MA, et al. The effect of physiotherapy on shoulder function in patients surgically treated for breast cancer: a randomised study. Acta Oncol. 2009;95:314–20.
28. Wanga T, Xub D, Liao Z. Anaphylactic reactions to isosulfan blue dye during sentinel lymph node biopsy for breast cancer. J Curr Surg. 2018;8:32–4.
29. Montgomery LL, Thorne AC, Van Zee KJ, et al. IB dye reactions during SLN mapping for breast cancer. Anesth Analg. 2002;95:385–8.
30. MacNeill F. New start: the UK SLNB training programme, a progress report. Ann R Coll Surg Engl (Suppl). 2007;89:60–1.
31. Wohrl S, Focke M, Hinterhuber G, Stingl G, Binder M. Near-fatal anaphylaxis to patent blue V. Br J Dermatol. 2004;150:1037–8.
32. The Society of Hospital Epidemiology of America; The Association for Practitioners in Infection Control; the Centers for Disease Control; The Surgical Infection Society. Consensus paper on the surveillance of surgical wound infection. Infect Control Hosp Epidemiol. 1992;13:599–605.

33. De Gournay E, et al. Impact of sentinel node biopsy on long-term quality of line in breast cancer patients. Br J Cancer. 2013;109:2783–91.
34. Kuehn T, Klauss W, Darsow M, Regele S, Flock F, Maiterth C, Dahlbender R, Wendt I, Kreienberg R. Long-term morbidity following axillary dissection in breast cancer patients–clinical assessment, significance for life quality and the impact of demographic, oncologic and therapeutic factors. Breast Cancer Res Treat. 2000;64(3):275–86.
35. Kissin MW, Querci della Rovere G, Easton D, Westbury G. Risk of lymphoedema following the treatment of breast cancer. Br J Surg. 1986;73(7):580–4.

Pathology Examination and Reporting of Sentinel Lymph Nodes: What Is Optimum?

7

Anu Malhotra and Sarah Pinder

7.1 Introduction

Sentinel lymph node biopsy (SLNB) is now standard of care for patients with no axillary nodal metastasis identified clinically or radiologically pre-operatively, as nodal status remains one of the most important prognostic factors in invasive breast cancer. More recently, targeted axillary dissection (TAD) with SLNB has been shown to be valuable for patients with excellent/complete response to neo-adjuvant chemotherapy. Both SLNB and TAD specimens require thorough and careful handling and examination in the pathology laboratory in order to deliver accurate clinical results. We describe here the methods used in histopathology laboratories for the assessment of these specimens and suggestions for features to be included in histology reports.

Rather than at least 15, and typically more, lymph nodes from an axillary clearance, pathologists will receive on average 2 lymph nodes in a SLNB specimen. This gives them the opportunity to examine these lymph nodes more thoroughly and potentially using a variety of methods, both intra-operatively (e.g. by frozen section, imprint cytology examination or one-step nucleic acid amplification [OSNA]) or on the formalin-fixed paraffin embedded post-operative tissue (e.g. additional 'step-sections'/'levels' and/or immunohistochemistry [IHC]). Some of these techniques require significant laboratory time and resources, and it is, therefore, important to

A. Malhotra
Guy's and St Thomas' NHS Foundation Trust, London, UK
e-mail: Anu.Malhotra@gstt.nhs.uk

S. Pinder (✉)
Guy's and St Thomas' NHS Foundation Trust, London, UK

King's College London, London, UK
e-mail: sarah.pinder@kcl.ac.uk

Chintamani (ed.), *Sentinel Node Biopsy in Breast Cancer*,
https://doi.org/10.1007/978-81-322-3994-9_7

assess their value and consider the significance of the identification of low-volume disease. This latter has changed as a result of trials, such as ACOSOG Z0011 [1], with consequent implications for optimum pathological laboratory handling.

Pathologists classify metastatic disease into three main categories: macro-metastases (>2 mm) (Fig. 7.1), micro-metastasis (>0.2–2 mm) (Fig. 7.2) (both considered 'node-positive') and isolated tumour cell clusters (0.2 mm or less) (Fig. 7.3), which are regarded as 'node-negative' in the primary surgery setting but which have different implications in those women in receipt of neo-adjuvant chemotherapy (see below).

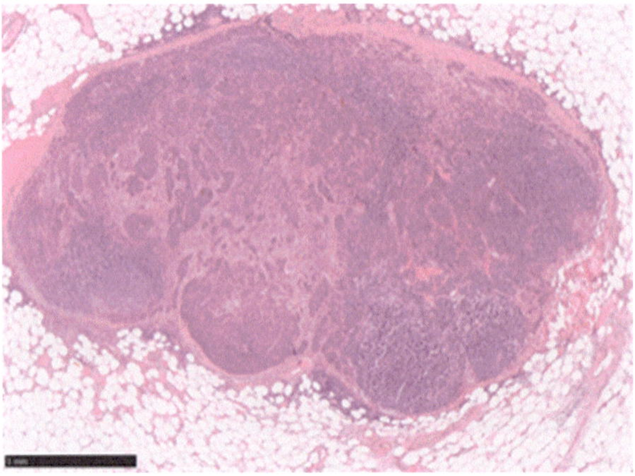

Fig. 7.1 Haematoxylin and eosin-stained section of lymph node almost entirely replaced by macro-metastatic carcinoma (i.e. >2 mm)

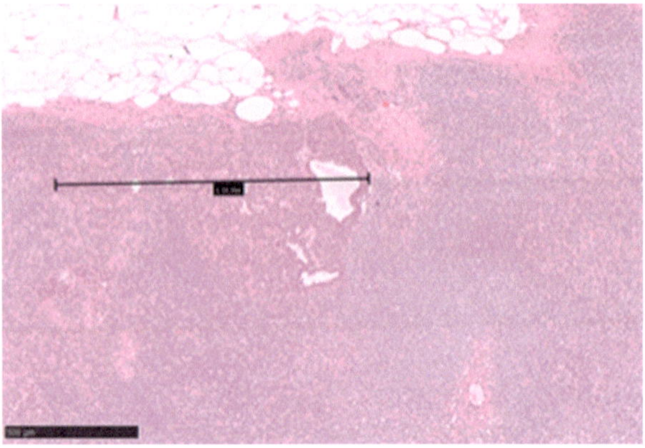

Fig. 7.2 Haematoxylin and eosin-stained section of lymph node with a focus of micro-metastatic carcinoma (i.e. >0.2 mm–2 mm)

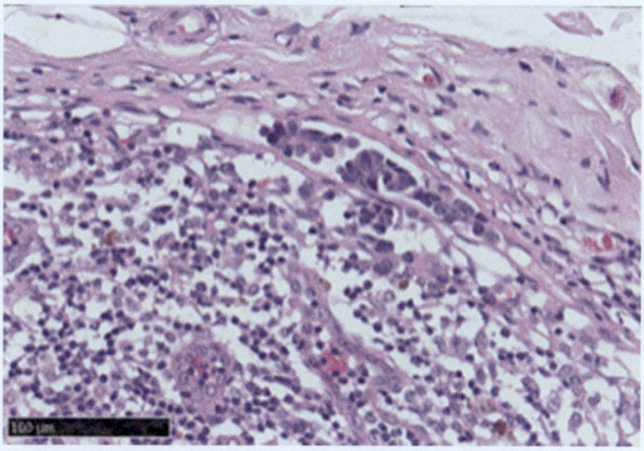

Fig. 7.3 Haematoxylin and eosin-stained section of lymph node with rather papillary clusters of cells in the sub-capsular sinus. This focus is 0.2 mm or less and therefore represents isolated tumour cell cluster (ITC)

7.2 Intra-operative Methods

Intra-operative assessment of lymph nodes allows patients with metastatic disease to undergo immediate axillary clearance rather than as a second procedure. However, this approach has been increasingly questioned for those with low-volume disease, and whilst intra-operative frozen section (FS) examination had been relatively widely utilised, its use has declined [2]. FS has, in experienced hands with diagnostic expertise, a high sensitivity and specificity, e.g. sensitivity of 92.6% and specificity of 100% in some series [3]. What is clear, and unsurprising, is that FS is better at the detection of macro-metastases than micro-metastases, or indeed ITCs; false-negative rates of 79.3% for ITCs, 59.8% for micro-metastasis and only 3.1% for macro-metastatic disease have been reported [4].

Like FS, imprint cytology requires technical and interpretive expertise but can be successfully used intra-operatively for SLN examination; in one recent series, the sensitivity in detecting metastases was 52.7% [49.7–55.8], the specificity was 99.5% [98.8–99.8], and the PPV and NPV were 97.3% [96.1–98.2] and 85.9% respectively [5]. As might be anticipated, similar to FS, imprint cytology is more accurate for the detection of larger-volume (i.e. macro-metastatic) disease.

OSNA involves the measurement of cytokeratin19 mRNA copy number in homogenised samples of the SLN. This has a higher sensitivity in detecting micro-metastases than FS or imprint cytology and an accuracy similar to FS and cytology for the identification of macro-metastases. It is an accurate method for intra-operative detection of metastases in the lymph nodes of patients with invasive breast cancer [6]. However, as the tissue has been homogenised, further histological assessment is not possible; other (e.g. non-metastatic) diseases cannot be diagnosed, the presence of extracapsular spread cannot be determined, and some false positives will very rarely result from, for example, benign epithelial inclusions. Whilst some groups use this technique satisfactorily, the methodology also takes longer than either FS or imprint cytology, and it is more expensive. Specifically, it is not recommended in the post-neo-adjuvant setting.

There are several reasons why the value of intra-operative assessment has been questioned in recent years. Imaging techniques for radiological assessment of the axilla have improved [7]. As a result, those patients most appropriate for axillary lymph node dissection (ALND) have already been identified pre-operatively with imaging and fine-needle aspiration cytology or core biopsy. Those with 'missed' nodal metastasis by imaging and cytology/core biopsy (i.e. only identified post-operatively) are typically neither extensive nor bulky disease. This is important because whilst ALND was traditionally advised for all breast cancer patients with positive lymph nodes, for the purposes of accurate staging of the axilla and loco-regional control, trials have demonstrated safety of omitting ALND in some patients (i.e. those with relatively low-volume disease). For these reasons, some groups now omit intra-operative assessment and recommend fixation and 'routine' processing post-operatively of the sentinel lymph nodes.

7.3 Post-operative Assessment

After immediate fixation in 10% buffered formalin, the lymph nodes are sliced as thinly as possible (2 mm or less), and all pieces are embedded and processed in paraffin wax, in one or more cassettes. Multiple pieces of a single SLN may be placed in one cassette or, if large, multiple cassettes, but each node must be separately embedded. A 3- to 4-μm-thick section is then cut from each block, and an haematoxylin and eosin (H&E)-stained section is examined; this approach facilitates the identification of the vast majority of macro-metastases (i.e. 2 mm or more) and is recommended in national guidelines (e.g. Royal College of Pathologists of GB and Ireland [https://www.rcpath.org/uploads/assets/7763be1c-d330-40e8-95d08f955752792a/G148_BreastDataset-hires-Jun16.pdf] and the College of American Pathologists [https://documents.cap.org/protocols/cp-breast-invasive-resection-20-4400.pdf]). The quality of the H&E stain is important to facilitate accurate diagnosis. Over and above one H&E section from each block, other options are utilised routinely by some; these include further H&E sections from the tissue deeper in the paraffin wax block (also called 'step-sections' or 'levels') and/or IHC. These approaches will particularly enable the detection of micro-metastases and ITCs (Fig. 7.3). Whilst some series have shown that these smaller deposits of carcinoma in the nodes are prognostic in patients with SLNBs that were negative on initial H&E examination, the difference in outcome at 5 years was small (1.2%), indicating that such further tests are not especially valuable [8], particularly, as noted above, when the need for further axillary treatment in this situation has been questioned.

IHC for cytokeratin markers, which are present in epithelial cells but not in lymphocytes, makes the identification of small foci of tumour in the lymph nodes easier, but it rarely facilitates the diagnosis of macro-metastases that are not visible on

Table 7.1 Features to be included in histopathology reports from SLN and TAD specimens

Number of nodes received	*N* =
Number 'positive'	Number with macro-metastasis, *N* =
	Number with micro-metastasis, *N* =
	Number with isolated tumour cell clusters, *N* =
Presence of extranodal spread[a]	Yes/no
Extent of extranodal spread	
Size of the largest lymph node metastasis	In mm
If neo-adjuvant specimen, number of nodes with reactive features that indicate metastasis was present previously	*N* =
If TAD, is marker clip site present?	Yes/no

[a]Extranodal spread has been shown to be a poor prognostic factor, particularly in those with 1–3 positive lymph nodes [Bucci JA, Kennedy CW, Burn J, Gillett DJ, Carmalt HL, Donnellan MJ, Joseph MG, Pendlebury SC. Implications of extranodal spread in node positive breast cancer: a review of survival and local recurrence. Breast. 2001 Jun;10(3):213–9. doi: 10.1054/brst.2000.0233. PMID: 14965587]

H&E stains. In one series of 216 patients, 56 (26%) had metastasis identified on H&E, IHC with Cam5.2 detected deposits in a further 9 (4%), but 4 (2%) had micro-metastasis, 5 (2%) had ITCs only, and none had macro-metastatic disease [9]. On re-review in this series, all the micro-metastases were visible on H&E sections; in other words, IHC did not add value to the careful examination of a high-quality H&E. Some groups recommend assessment of IHC in cases known to be potentially difficult to identify such as in invasive lobular carcinoma and/or cases of post-neo-adjuvant chemotherapy with good response (see below). The UK reporting guidelines suggest that IHC may be performed when there are cells suspected as carcinoma but do not recommend H&E levels or IHC as routine (https://www.rcpath.org/uploads/assets/7763be1c-d330-40e8-95d08f955752792a/G148_BreastDataset-hires-Jun16.pdf). It should, however, be noted that in our own department, three H&E levels are examined, partly to compensate for a potentially uneven first H&E section and for tissue slices that may be >2-mm thick, and this is a widespread practice. Histology reports include the features shown in Table 7.1.

7.4 Targeted Axillary Dissection and SLB Post-Neo-adjuvant Chemotherapy (NACT)

Assessment of the SLNB from patients deemed to be node-negative pre-treatment before systemic therapy, and remaining so, clinically/radiologically is not different from those who have not received NACT. Assessment of those with known node metastases (e.g. by pre-operative imaging and core biopsy) who have had good response to therapy is, however, often more difficult. Macroscopically the targeted lymph node bearing marker clip typically shows fibrosis as a response to its insertion; this may thus feel firm and even enlarged grossly, even if no metastasis was/is present. Of note, pathologists should record that the marker clip site is present to confirm appropriate excision has been achieved. The targeted node and additional SLNs should be sliced at 2 mm or less intervals and all embedded, as for those patients who have not received systemic therapy pre-operatively.

Microscopically, when there is response to NACT, there is typically reactive fibrosis in the node, sometimes along with other histological features such as sheets of foamy macrophages. These changes may mask any scattered residual carcinoma that may be difficult to recognise and may potentially be missed if great care is not taken in examination. Such occasional cases may benefit from IHC with cytokeratins for definitive diagnosis and confirmation of their epithelial nature. In particular, the importance of low-volume disease (micro-metastasis or ITCs) is different in the post-NACT setting as low-volume disease may potentially represent response to treatment of larger foci. Both micrometastases and ITCs are considered node-positive post-NACT; this may potentially be confusing when reporting the TNM stage, and it should be noted that pN0(i+) (i.e. without prior systemic therapy) is not equivalent to ypN0(i+) (i.e. post-NACT).

Microscopic measurement, and thus categorisation, of small residual foci post-NACT may also not be straightforward; whilst the AJCC TNM staging manual states that the largest focus of residual carcinoma in the lymph nodes is used for ypN categorisation, others, including ourselves, record the residual cancer burden (RCB) score in our reports [10]. We therefore record the largest extent of carcinoma cells including intervening stromal fibrosis as the metastatic size. In addition, in the post-NACT setting, as well as the total number of nodes removed, the number with residual metastasis, the size of the largest focus and the presence of extranodal spread, we report the number of nodes with treatment-related fibrosis, both with and without residual viable carcinoma. This may be helpful in conjunction with pre-treatment imaging to determine the number involved with metastatic tumour before systemic therapy, which may assist in making decisions regarding the extent of subsequent radiotherapy.

In conclusion, the goal posts continue to change for pathological assessment and reporting of SLNs. The value of intra-operative assessment, if high-quality imaging and cytology/core biopsy are available, is more questionable than previously, as most patients who are not identified as having nodal metastasis pre-operatively will have low-volume disease and will not benefit from axillary node dissection. The aim of the pathologist should be to apply a methodology that identifies all cases with macro-metastatic tumour in the SLN in those who have not received neo-adjuvant therapy; slicing as thinly as possible with a high-quality H&E section is advised, and an exhaustive search for micrometastasis and ITC metastatic disease is not clinically valuable. In the post-NACT setting, however, assessment can be more difficult; the gross handling of specimens should be the same, but histological examination may sometimes warrant IHC, as well as good quality, thin H&E sections, to accurately identify and measure small foci of residual disease, such as ITCs, which are regarded as node-positive post-NACT.

References

1. Axillary dissection on 10-year overall survival among women with invasive breast cancer and sentinel node metastasis: the ACOSOG Z0011 (Alliance) randomized clinical trial. JAMA. 2017;318(10):918–26. https://doi.org/10.1001/jama.2017.11470. PMID: 28898379; PMCID: PMC5672806.
2. Jorns JM, Kidwell KM. Sentinel lymph node frozen-section utilization declines after publication of American College of Surgeons oncology group Z0011 trial results with no change in subsequent surgery for axillary lymph node dissection. Am J Clin Pathol. 2016;146(1):57–66. https://doi.org/10.1093/ajcp/aqw078. Epub 2016 Jul 3. PMID: 27373347.
3. Somashekhar SP, Naikoo ZA, Zaveri SS, Holla S, Chandra S, Mishra S, Parameswaran RV. Intraoperative frozen section evaluation of sentinel lymph nodes in breast carcinoma: single-institution Indian experience. Indian J Surg. 2015;77(Suppl 2):335–40. https://doi.org/10.1007/s12262-013-0827-2. Epub 2013 Feb 5. PMID: 26730021; PMCID: PMC4692900.
4. Wong J, Yong WS, Thike AA, Iqbal J, Salahuddin AS, Ho GH, Madhukumar P, Tan BK, Ong KW, Tan PH. False negative rate for intraoperative sentinel lymph node frozen section in patients with breast cancer: a retrospective analysis of patients in a single Asian institution. J Clin Pathol. 2015;68(7):536–40. https://doi.org/10.1136/jclinpath-2014-202799. Epub 2015 Apr 8. PMID: 25855801.
5. Iacuzzo C, Scomersi S, Giudici F, Bonadio L, Troian M, Bellio G, Rizzardi C, Bonazza D, Zanconati F, Bortul M. The current role of touch imprint cytology in sentinel lymph node intraoperatory examination. Breast J. 2020;26(3):576–7. https://doi.org/10.1111/tbj.13619. Epub 2019 Sep 4. PMID: 31486216.
6. Shi F, Liang Z, Zhang Q, Wang C, Liu X. The performance of one-step nucleic acid amplification assay for intraoperative detection of sentinel lymph node macrometastasis in breast cancer: an updated meta-analysis. Breast. 2018;39:39–45. https://doi.org/10.1016/j.breast.2018.03.005. Epub 2018 Mar 22. PMID: 29574393.
7. Lowes S, Leaver A, Cox K, Satchithananda K, Cosgrove D, Lim A. Evolving imaging techniques for staging axillary lymph nodes in breast cancer. Clin Radiol. 2018;73(4):396–409. https://doi.org/10.1016/j.crad.2018.01.003. Epub 2018 Feb 10. PMID: 29439780.
8. Weaver DL, Ashikaga T, Krag DN, Skelly JM, Anderson SJ, Har-low SP, Julian TB, Mamounas EP, Wolmark N. Effect of occult metastases on survival in node-negative breast cancer. N Engl J Med. 2011;364:412–21. https://doi.org/10.1056/NEJMoa1008108.
9. Klevesath MB, Bobrow LG, Pinder SE, Purushotham AD. The value of immunohistochemistry in sentinel lymph node histopathology in breast cancer. Br J Cancer. 2005;92(12):2201–5. https://doi.org/10.1038/sj.bjc.6602641. PMID: 15942633; PMCID: PMC2361824.
10. Symmans WF, Peintinger F, Hatzis C, Rajan R, Kuerer H, Valero V, Assad L, Poniecka A, Hennessy B, Green M, Buzdar AU, Singletary SE, Hortobagyi GN, Pusztai L. Measurement of residual breast cancer burden to predict survival after neoadjuvant chemotherapy. J Clin Oncol. 2007;25(28):4414–22. https://doi.org/10.1200/JCO.2007.10.6823. Epub 2007 Sep 4. PMID: 17785706.

8 Newer Modalities for the Detection and Assessment of the Sentinel Lymph Node

Andreas Karakatsanis and Ashutosh Kothari

8.1 Background

The combination of radioactive colloid (RI, Tc^{99}) with a blue dye (BD) for visual reference has traditionally been regarded as the gold standard for the mapping and identification of sentinel lymph nodes (SLNs), following the first landmark trials validating the outcomes of SLN biopsy (SLNB) [1–4]. The isotope is usually injected in the sub-areolar region or in the parenchyma around the tumour, a few hours before the operation. The BD is injected intra-operatively under anaesthesia, and the breast is massaged to facilitate tracer migration towards the axilla. The tracers reach the SLN via the lymphatic system. The SLN is then detected using a hand-held gamma probe or by following a blue lymphatic to a blue SLN. The procedure is conventionally considered complete when the residual gamma probe signal in the axilla is less than 10% of the maximum signal of the lymph node retrieved [4]. This technique results in detection rates as high as 99% with a false-negative rate of less than 5% and axillary recurrence rates lower than 2% [5–7]. The procedure is reasonably intuitive, is easy to standardise and has therefore gained wide acceptance. This combined technique over time has become the benchmark or the reference for SLNB procedures.

There are, however, some drawbacks and limitations. The use of RI requires a nuclear medicine department, or, at best, access to local nuclear medicine facilities.

A. Karakatsanis (✉)
Department of Surgical Sciences, Uppsala University, Uppsala, Sweden

Section for Breast Surgery, Department of Surgery, Uppsala University Hospital, Uppsala, Sweden

A. Kothari
Department of Breast Surgery, Guy's & St Thomas' NHS Foundation Trust, London, UK

King's College, London, UK

Chintamani (ed.), *Sentinel Node Biopsy in Breast Cancer*,
https://doi.org/10.1007/978-81-322-3994-9_8

The legislations that regulate the handling and disposal of radioactive material are complicated and rigid. Despite the radiation doses being very small, repeated exposure may confer possible health hazards and stress for both patients and staff. The short half-life (6 h) of Technetium 99 m (Tc) limits its usefulness as it needs to be administered on the day of surgery, or, at most, the afternoon before, incurring more cost for a higher dose to ensure detectable axillary activity. This leads to logistic issues that may cause avoidable stress to patients on the day of their surgery. Finally, ease of access to the RI seems to be a challenge, especially in the global setting. Recent data from the World Health Organization indicated that only 60% of patients in developed countries have access to the procedure, with this figure dropping down to 5% in China and even lower in the rest of the world [8]. On the other hand, the BD is allergenic, and severe anaphylactic reactions have been reported in around 0.1% of patients. This is why BD is administered after the induction of anaesthesia so that vital functions are monitored. The injection and massage for 5–10 min that are routinely performed for tracer migration prolong the duration of the procedure. In addition, the injection of BD may cause skin staining that has been shown to persist in up to 42% of patients for up to 2 years post-surgery [9, 10]. These issues underline the clinical need for non-radioactive, non-allergenic alternative tracers comparable with the current benchmarks.

8.2 What Should an Optimal Method Look Like?

Surgical techniques need to be both pragmatic and flexible at the same time. This suggests that novel tracers should provide at least equivalent outcomes in terms of performance and at the same time negate the inherent drawbacks of the dual technique. Ideally, novel tracers should be able to meet new tailored patient-specific clinical needs and scenarios.

In summary, a novel tracer should provide the following:

- Comparable (or better) detection rate
- Comparable (or less) adverse effects
- Easier logistics, unhindered access, potential for use in the global setting
- Ability to address tailored patient scenarios

8.3 Novel Techniques for Axillary Mapping

Research has focused on two different concepts for the optimal surgical evaluation of the axillary nodal status. First is the use of non-radioactive tracers that perform comparably to the combination of RI and BD. Second is the use of methods that represent a hybrid approach between minimally invasive and non-invasive imaging techniques. Finally, the use of alternative non-invasive approaches based on tumour biology, aiming to develop predictive nomograms through validation cohorts. More recently, artificial intelligence, machine learning and artificial neural networks have been described with varying results. However, they have not gained broad acceptance and exceed the scope of the present chapter.

8.4 Indocyanine Green (ICG)

The use of indocyanine green (ICG) as a tracer for identifying sentinel nodes has been extensively investigated since 2005, and interest has increased in recent years. The majority of studies come from Asia, but several European groups have also investigated the technique and its outcomes. Other applications in breast surgery include but are not limited to the assessment of flap perfusion in reconstructive surgery and axillary reverse mapping to preserve lymphatics of the upper extremity during axillary dissection and for the identification of chest wall perforators. ICG binds to plasma proteins after a subdermal/intradermal injection in the retroareolar or peri-areolar area. This results in a high concentration of dye in the lymphatics. Currently, there are different apparatuses used for visualisation [PDE: photodynamic eye (Hamamatsu, Japan)) The medical imaging projection system (MIPS, Panasonic Japan), HyperEye system (Mizuho, Japan)], that are all based on the principle of fluorescence.

- Technique

  The studies on ICG are at best heterogeneous, not only in relation to the dose and concentration of ICG but also the site and depth of injection. Most studies, however, discuss injection in the peri-areolar/sub-areolar area. ICG has a half-life of as low as 3–4 min, which translates to a time window of between 20 and 30 min when the dye is identifiable [11–31]. This implies that ICG is best administered intra-operatively, although the dose may be repeated. However, if the lymphatics are transected, then this poses a concern of "leakage" that could potentially disturb the surgical field and identification. It provides the benefit of real-time transcutaneous lymphography, but the maximum depth for localization is 1.5–2 cm. A high body mass index is a limitation in some studies, as a negative correlation has been noticed for detection rates in patients with a BMI > 40.

  After tracer injection and migration in the axilla, SLNB is conducted by using fluorescence, and all fluorescent lymph nodes are identified under near infrared (NIR) imaging and removed.
- Outcomes

  The performance of ICG has been extensively tested in different study designs [11–34]. In studies with paired design, it has been found to outperform BD and to be non-inferior to the radioisotope with or without BD. Most citing studies and meta-analyses show a detection rate of over 97%, whereas single-arm cohort studies reproduce similar findings. As previously mentioned, ICG has been tested in different concentrations, injection volumes and injection sites, without a considerable variance in outcomes. There is, however, data that suggests that a higher concentration and smaller volume correlate with SLNB sensitivity. At the same time, it has been shown that high concentration in the lymph node is associated with higher fluorescence intensity.

Other studies from the Netherlands have proposed the combination of the ICG and the radioisotope as well as the use of conjugated tracers combining radioactivity and fluorescence [32, 34]. These, however, have not provided consistent findings and have not demonstrated any benefit from combining the tracers. Additionally, the numbers are small, and in the absence of a clear benefit, these alternatives have not been adopted in routine practice.

Regarding the number of SLNs retrieved, the original studies suggested that many more nodes were identified and retrieved with a median of five SLNs, which suggested more extensive dissection in the axilla. Some authors were quite concerned about this. More recent studies do not show any difference; however, the majority of published data suggests that ICG yields more SLNs than the combination of isotope and BD, or each tracer separately. Further analyses suggest that this is a finding that reflects study design and quality, rather than a limitation of the method. However, surgeons should be conscious of this when using the technique.

In summary, ICG is an effective tracer in terms of detection, with a very credible safety profile, an incidence of adverse effects <1:10,000 and without any serious adverse events being reported. The need for NIR imaging systems, the need for a separate technique for occult lesion localisation and the lack of health-economy data should be taken into consideration before the adoption of the technique.

8.5 Superparamagnetic Iron Oxide Nanoparticles (SPIO)

Superparamagnetic iron oxide nanoparticles (SPIO) have a size of approximately 59–60 nm and have a dextran coating. This allows for their retention within the cells of the reticuloendothelial systems, predominantly, macrophages. Subsequently, the sequestrated iron is metabolised after iron homeostasis. It was originally used as an intravenous contrast agent for liver MRI scans, and its use as an SLN tracer has been investigated over the last 10 years. Currently, there are two available magnetic probes (SentiMag, Endomag, UK and TAKUMI, Tokyo University), and they are used with the SPIOs Magtrace© and Resovist©, respectively.

- Technique

  The initial studies published largely involved the peri-operative or intra-operative administration of SPIO [35–47]. The tracer was injected in the subareolar region, followed by a 5-min massage to promote lymphatic migration to the axilla. The time required for migration of the tracer is 20 min but has been reported to be as high as 1 h. However, one should allow for a minimum of 20 min from injection and massage to SLNB. A negative correlation between patient BMI and transcutaneous detection has been demonstrated; reassuringly, however, after the axillary incision, high BMI does not seem to hinder SLN detection [41]. After the SPIO injection, SLNs are identified by using a special handheld probe, and the nodes with the highest concentration of magnetised SPIO are removed. SPIO also discolours the sentinel nodes to a deep grey-brown colour and in doing so also facilitates visual identification. At the time of writing, SPIO is the only tracer available with this unique dual identification property, whereas lower doses than the original 2 ml have been successfully tested [47, 48].

SPIO seems to linger at the injection site and within the SLN for prolonged periods, which allows for its administration days to weeks before the intended surgical intervention. This provides flexibility in planning, improved logistics and more efficient theatre scheduling. Preclinical data suggest that the concentration of SPIO in the SLNs reaches a plateau at 24 h post interstitial administration, and clinical studies have shown successful SLN identification up to 6 months [49].

The peri-areolar injection of SPIO in the breast results in a brownish cutaneous discolouration in patients that undergo breast-conserving therapy. However, studies suggest that a lower-volume peri-areolar/sub-areolar injection results in lesser discolouration. Deeper, peri-tumoural and intraparenchymal injection also result in significantly less staining whilst retaining a very high detection rate and accuracy. In a large, patient-level meta-analysis, a lower dose of 1 mL injected peri-tumourally 1–7 days before surgery resulted in excellent detection rates whilst retaining similar concordance rates with the isotope [50]. This demonstrates that SPIO is a tracer that can be administered flexibly without affecting outcomes.

– Outcomes

The performance of SPIO has been extensively tested since 2013 in different study designs. Most studies have a paired design, with patients being their own controls and were designed to demonstrate non-inferiority. In these studies, SPIO has constantly performed comparably to the isotope with detection rates >97%, and non-inferiority has formally been established in meta-analyses. Single-arm cohort studies have also reproduced similar findings. SPIO has been tested in different doses (2 ml in 3 ml of dilutant, 2 ml, 1.5 ml, 1 ml and 0.5 ml undiluted), different injection sites and different timings of injection (peri-operative or pre-operative). In all these scenarios, there is no clinically relevant difference in outcomes when it comes to successful SLN detection [49]. Until the present day, there are no studies that have investigated hybrid SPIO-based tracers or the combination of SPIO with another visual tracer for SLN detection. Given the fact that SPIO is a dual tracer per se, one could argue against the need for such studies.

Initial studies suggested that SPIO yields more SLNs, but this finding has not been confirmed in later single-arm studies or head-to-head comparisons. Even in cumulative analyses, pooled values are comparable with no more than two to three SLNs excised (crude mean 1.93 nodes vs 1.85 for isotope with or without BD) [50]. Looking into the literature, several authors point to the fact that this may be explained by overlapping bias [41]. This implies that when SPIO and radioisotope were co-administered, SLNs that were registered as magnetic either had a very low signal and were primarily detected with the isotope or the lack of familiarity with the technique together with diffuse magnetic signal in the axilla may have led to the excision of extra tissue. However, SPIO results in magnetic and coloured lymph nodes that can be identified and excised without excessive tissue removal, suggesting that the surgeon should take advantage of these properties to avoid unnecessary dissection.

8.5.1 Extended Timeframe and the SentiNot Procedure

The fact that SPIO lingers in the tissue for prolonged periods has allowed for the exploration of a pre-operative injection over a wider timeframe. First results indicated safe and accurate SLN detection up to 27 days before surgery. Subsequently, the SentiNot procedure was developed [49]. In patients with a pre-operative diagnosis of pure DCIS, SPIO was injected in the breast on the day of breast surgery to mark the SLN. No axillary surgery was performed at that point. After definitive specimen pathology, only patients with an upgrade to invasive cancer underwent delayed SLNB with the concomitant use of radioisotope. This technique ensured that all patients with pure DCIS avoided unnecessary axillary surgery, corresponding to 78% of the study cohort. In patients that underwent the SentiNot procedure, a median of 47 days after primary surgery, SPIO performed better than the combination radioisotope and BD, with a detection rate exceeding 95%, regardless of whether breast-conserving therapy or mastectomy had been performed [51]. The technique is currently investigated in a large-scale randomised controlled trial to support the de-escalation of axillary surgery in low-risk settings. At the same time, the role of delayed SLNB in the setting of primary systemic therapy is being investigated.

Looking into the safety profile, no serious adverse effects have been reported from the use of SPIO. The main concerns associated with its use are susceptibility artefacts in post-operative breast MRI and skin staining. Early reports of artefacts showed extended susceptibility artefacts after sub-areolar injection of 2 ml of SPIO with 3 ml of dilutant, persisting up to 4 years and affecting the interpretation of the breast MRI scan. Following this, low-volume and non-dedicated studies have reported similar results. The Uppsala group made the early observation that a peritumoural injection is associated with less skin staining and, possibly, since the bulk of SPIO is removed with the tumour specimen, fewer MRI artefacts. Whilst clinical MRIs performed were in line with this observation, the hypothesis is currently being tested in a prospective study with planned follow-up of up to 5 years to accumulate robust data. More recently, a Dutch group reported no artefacts after the intratumoral injection of SPIO, but the small numbers in this study do not allow for a definitive conclusion [50]. It is evident, however, that injecting the SPIO within the breast parenchyma to be excised seems to be a reasonable approach in dealing with the prevention of these problems. To put this matter into context, it should not be forgotten that post-operative breast MRI has little or no role in routine mammographic surveillance of women with non-hereditary breast cancer treated with breast conservation.

Skin staining is also associated with the residual SPIO at the injection site, and outcomes from literature have shown skin staining as high as 84% following breast conservation, with a median prevalence of 30%. In long-term follow-up, peri-tumoural injection and a lower dose have constantly been associated with much lower skin staining rates (as low as 8.6%) that are smaller in size and paler in intensity [50].

In terms of health economics, the use of SPIO has been validated in studies from Sweden and Germany. Despite the differences in the healthcare settings and patient pathways, these studies showed that SPIO may yield beneficial effects in health economics, resources and patient satisfaction [50]. Another perceived advantage for SPIO is that the same probe is used to detect the SLN as well as the occult breast lesions marked with paramagnetic seeds, allowing for the use of a single integrated magnetic platform.

8.6 Minimally Invasive Approaches in SLN Mapping

The use of contrast-enhanced ultrasound (CEUS) with microbubbles has yielded interesting results [52, 53]. A contrast agent (e.g. SonoVue®; SonazoidTM; Daiichi Sankyo Japan) consisting of a phospholipid shell that contains microbubbles of sulphur hexafluoride gas (SF6) is injected intradermally in the areola. Subsequently, an axillary CEUS is used to identify axillary lymph nodes with contrast uptake that are, by definition, the sentinel nodes. This is a method that can be used pre-operatively to conduct a fine needle aspiration (FNAC) or core biopsy before performing the surgical SLNB. The larger body of evidence stems either from dedicated centres that have familiarity with the technique or small case series, often without a control group [54–72]. More studies are needed to standardise the technique and improve the sensitivity that was shown to be as low as 54% (pooled value, 95% CI 47–61%) in a recent review. On the other hand, the procedure has a very high specificity [100% (pooled)]. No adverse reactions have been documented, but there remains a theoretical possibility for hypersensitivity reactions. Pre-operative identification and localisation range between 70 and 100%. The main advantage of this method is the absence of radiation. However, when compared with ICG and SPIO, network meta-analyses suggest that the procedure does not perform comparably [73].

Another novel method used is computed tomographic lymphography (CTLG). It has been used pre-operatively to predict lymph node metastasis. In the CTLG, an iodine contrast (iopamidol) is used, and SLNB is then performed with BD or ICG [74]. A detection rate of 98 = 100% has been reported when done pre-operatively and reaches 100% when combined with CTLG-assisted biopsy. The false-negative and false-positive rates for macro-metastases have been reported to be high, 17.9% and 16.4%, which suggest lower diagnostic accuracy. Other disadvantages include the lack of standardisation, X-ray radiation and risk of allergic reactions when using iodine contrast. The advantages are high detection rate and no need for radioactive tracers.

Recent studies have investigated the combination of axillary CTLG and MRI lymphography after SPIO injection in the breast. In two reports from Japan, the procedure yielded a remarkably high diagnostic accuracy in 3 Tesla MRI cameras, in T2 sequences with water exaltation [75]. However, the procedure is costly and requires increased resources, which poses a challenge to its wider acceptance. Finally, the combination of SPIO-MRI lymphography and magnetic probe-guided ultrasound for transcutaneous SLN biopsy has been recently presented. In the MagUS trial, SPIO MRI lymphography allowed for the localisation of axillary SLNs [76]. Subsequently, an axillary ultrasound was performed with magnetic probe guidance. When a node was identified in the area of maximum transcutaneous signal, a core biopsy was performed, and the retrieved tissue was assessed for brown discolouration and magnetic signal. The outcome was compared with the surgical SLNB. In this phase 2 trial, the MagUS procedure was performed with much higher accuracy than the standard ultrasound (AUC 95.5 vs 50.5, $p < 0.001$) and staged the axilla with comparable accuracy to that of SLNB. This data, albeit promising, need to be further evaluated in larger trials before routine implementation.

References

1. Umberto V, et al. A randomized comparison of sentinel-node biopsy with routine axillary dissection in breast cancer. N Engl J Med. 2003;349:546.
2. Krag DN, et al. Sentinel-lymph-node resection compared with conventional axillary-lymph-node dissection in clinically node-negative patients with breast cancer: overall survival findings from the NSABP B-32 randomised phase 3 trial. Lancet Oncol. 2010;11:927–33.
3. Mansel RE, et al. Randomized multicenter trial of sentinel node biopsy versus standard axillary treatment in operable breast cancer: the ALMANAC trial. J Natl Cancer Inst. 2006;98:599–609.
4. Krag D, et al. The sentinel node in breast cancer--a multicenter validation study. N Engl J Med. 1998;339:941–6.
5. Giuliano AE, et al. Axillary dissection vs no axillary dissection in women with invasive breast cancer and sentinel node metastasis: a randomized clinical trial. JAMA. 2011;305:569–75.
6. Bergkvist L, Frisell J. Multicentre validation study of sentinel node biopsy for staging in breast cancer. Br J Surg. 2005;92:1221–4.
7. Donker M, et al. Radiotherapy or surgery of the axilla after a positive sentinel node in breast cancer (EORTC 10981-22023 AMAROS): a randomised, multicentre, open-label, phase 3 non-inferiority trial. Lancet Oncol. 2014;15:1303–10.
8. WHO. Breast cancer: prevention and control. WHO http://www.who.int/cancer/detection/breastcancer/en/.
9. Barthelmes L, et al. Adverse reactions to patent blue V dye - the NEW START and ALMANAC experience. Eur J Surg Oncol. 2010;36:399–403.
10. Masannat Y, Shenoy H, Speirs V, Hanby A, Horgan K. Properties and characteristics of the dyes injected to assist axillary sentinel node localization in breast surgery. Eur J Surg Oncol. 2006;32:381–4.
11. Samorani D, et al. The use of indocyanine green to detect sentinel nodes in breast cancer: a prospective study. Eur J Surg Oncol J. 2015;41:64–70.
12. Wishart GC, Loh S-W, Jones L, Benson JR. A feasibility study (ICG-10) of indocyanine green (ICG) fluorescence mapping for sentinel lymph node detection in early breast cancer. Eur J Surg Oncol. 2012;38:651–6.

13. Ballardini B, et al. The indocyanine green method is equivalent to the 99mTc-labeled radiotracer method for identifying the sentinel node in breast cancer: a concordance and validation study. Eur J Surg Oncol J. 2013;39:1332–6.
14. Hojo T, Nagao T, Kikuyama M, Akashi S, Kinoshita T. Evaluation of sentinel node biopsy by combined fluorescent and dye method and lymph flow for breast cancer. Breast. 2010;19:210–3.
15. Murawa D, Hirche C, Dresel S, Hünerbein M. Sentinel lymph node biopsy in breast cancer guided by indocyanine green fluorescence. Br J Surg. 2009;96:1289–94.
16. Polom K, Murawa D, Nowaczyk P, Rho YS, Murawa P. Breast cancer sentinel lymph node mapping using near infrared guided indocyanine green and indocyanine green--human serum albumin in comparison with gamma emitting radioactive colloid tracer. Eur J Surg Oncol. 2012;38:137–42.
17. Sugie T, et al. Evaluation of the clinical utility of the ICG fluorescence method compared with the radioisotope method for sentinel lymph node biopsy in breast cancer. Ann Surg Oncol. 2016;23:44–50.
18. Papathemelis T, et al. Sentinel lymph node biopsy in breast cancer patients by means of Indocyanine green using the Karl Storz VITOM® fluorescence camera. Biomed Res Int. 2018;2018:6251468.
19. Chang YW, et al. Sentinel lymph node detection using fluorescein and blue light-emitting diodes in patients with breast carcinoma: a single-center prospective study. Asian J Surg. 2020;43:220–6.
20. Mazouni C, et al. Prospective evaluation of the limitations of near-infrared imaging in detecting axillary sentinel lymph nodes in primary breast cancer. Breast J. 2018;24:1006–9.
21. Tagaya N, et al. Intraoperative identification of sentinel lymph nodes by near-infrared fluorescence imaging in patients with breast cancer. Am J Surg. 2008;195:850–3.
22. Toh U, et al. Navigation surgery for intraoperative sentinel lymph node detection using Indocyanine green (ICG) fluorescence real-time imaging in breast cancer. Breast Cancer Res Treat. 2015;153:337–44.
23. Tong M, Guo W, Gao W. Use of fluorescence imaging in combination with patent blue dye versus patent blue dye alone in sentinel lymph node biopsy in breast cancer. J Breast Cancer. 2014;17:250–5.
24. Abe H, et al. Indocyanine green fluorescence imaging system for sentinel lymph node biopsies in early breast cancer patients. Surg Today. 2011;41:197–202.
25. He K, et al. Comparison between the indocyanine green fluorescence and blue dye methods for sentinel lymph node biopsy using novel fluorescence image-guided resection equipment in different types of hospitals. Transl Res J Lab Clin Med. 2016;178:74–80.
26. Liu J, Huang L, Wang N, Chen P. Indocyanine green detects sentinel lymph nodes in early breast cancer. J Int Med Res. 2017;45:514–24.
27. Pitsinis V, Provenzano E, Kaklamanis L, Wishart GC, Benson JR. Indocyanine green fluorescence mapping for sentinel lymph node biopsy in early breast cancer. Surg Oncol. 2015;24:375–9.
28. Hokimoto N, et al. A novel color fluorescence navigation system for intraoperative transcutaneous lymphatic mapping and resection of sentinel lymph nodes in breast cancer: comparison with the combination of gamma probe scanning and visible dye methods. Oncology. 2018;94:99–106.
29. Guo W, et al. Breast cancer sentinel lymph node mapping using near-infrared guided indocyanine green in comparison with blue dye. Tumour Biol. 2014;35:3073–8.
30. Guo J, et al. Comparison of sentinel lymph node biopsy guided by indocyanine green, blue dye, and their combination in breast cancer patients: a prospective cohort study. World J Surg Oncol. 2017;15:196.
31. Hirano A, et al. A comparison of indocyanine green fluorescence imaging plus blue dye and blue dye alone for sentinel node navigation surgery in breast cancer patients. Ann Surg Oncol. 2012;19:4112–6.

32. Schaafsma BE, et al. Clinical trial of combined radio- and fluorescence-guided sentinel lymph node biopsy in breast cancer. Br J Surg. 2013;100:1037–44.
33. Valente SA, et al. Near infrared fluorescent lymph node mapping with Indocyanine green in breast cancer patients: a prospective trial. J Am Coll Surg. 2019;228:672–8.
34. Vermersch C, Raia-Barjat T, Chapelle C, Lima S, Chauleur C. Randomized comparison between indocyanine green fluorescence plus 99mtechnetium and 99mtechnetium alone methods for sentinel lymph node biopsy in breast cancer. Sci Rep. 2019;9:6943.
35. Shiozawa M, et al. Sentinel lymph node biopsy in patients with breast cancer using superparamagnetic iron oxide and a magnetometer. Breast Cancer. 2013;20:223–9.
36. Douek M, et al. Sentinel node biopsy using a magnetic tracer versus standard technique: the SentiMAG Multicentre Trial. Ann Surg Oncol. 2014;21:1237–45.
37. Rubio IT, et al. The superparamagnetic iron oxide is equivalent to the Tc99 radiotracer method for identifying the sentinel lymph node in breast cancer. Eur J Surg Oncol. 2015;41:46–51.
38. Thill M, et al. The Central-European SentiMag study: sentinel lymph node biopsy with superparamagnetic iron oxide (SPIO) vs. radioisotope. Breast. 2014;23:175–9.
39. Piñero-Madrona A, et al. Superparamagnetic iron oxide as a tracer for sentinel node biopsy in breast cancer: a comparative non-inferiority study. Eur J Surg Oncol. 2015;41:991–7.
40. Ghilli M, et al. The superparamagnetic iron oxide tracer: a valid alternative in sentinel node biopsy for breast cancer treatment. Eur J Cancer Care. 2017;26.
41. Karakatsanis A, et al. The Nordic SentiMag trial: a comparison of super paramagnetic iron oxide (SPIO) nanoparticles versus Tc(99) and patent blue in the detection of sentinel node (SN) in patients with breast cancer and a meta-analysis of earlier studies. Breast Cancer Res Treat. 2016;157:281–94.
42. Houpeau J-L, et al. Sentinel lymph node identification using superparamagnetic iron oxide particles versus radioisotope: the French Sentimag feasibility trial. J Surg Oncol. 2016;113:501–7.
43. Coufal O, Fait V, Lžičařová E, Chrenko V, Žaloudík J. [SentiMag--the magnetic detection system of sentinel lymph nodes in breast cancer]. Rozhl V Chir Mesicnik Ceskoslovenske Chir Spolecnosti. 2015;94:283–8.
44. Alvarado MD, et al. SentimagIC: a non-inferiority trial comparing superparamagnetic iron oxide versus technetium-99m and blue dye in the detection of axillary sentinel nodes in patients with early-stage breast cancer. Ann Surg Oncol. 2019;26:3510–6.
45. Hamzah JL, et al. A pilot study comparing Sentimag/Sienna versus standard modality for sentinel lymph node identification in patients with breast cancer. Breast J. 2020;26:1074–7.
46. Taruno K, et al. Multicenter clinical trial on sentinel lymph node biopsy using superparamagnetic iron oxide nanoparticles and a novel handheld magnetic probe. J Surg Oncol. 2019;120:1391–6.
47. Rubio IT, Rodriguez-Revuelto R, Espinosa-Bravo M, Siso C, Rivero J, Esgueva A. A randomized study comparing different doses of superparamagnetic iron oxide tracer for sentinel lymph node biopsy in breast cancer: the SUNRISE study. Eur J Surg Oncol. 2020;46:2195–201.
48. Hersi AF, et al. Optimizing dose and timing in magnetic tracer techniques for sentinel lymph node detection in early breast cancers: the prospective multicenter Sentidose trial. Cancers. 2021;13:693.
49. Karakatsanis A, et al. Effect of preoperative injection of superparamagnetic iron oxide particles on rates of sentinel lymph node dissection in women undergoing surgery for ductal carcinoma in situ (SentiNot study). Br J Surg. 2019;106:720–8.
50. Pantiora E, et al. Evolution and refinement of magnetically guided sentinel lymph node detection in breast cancer: meta-analysis. Br J Surg. 2023;110:410. https://doi.org/10.1093/bjs/znac426.
51. Karakatsanis A, et al. Delayed sentinel lymph node dissection in patients with a preoperative diagnosis of ductal cancer in situ by preoperative injection with superparamagnetic iron oxide (SPIO) nanoparticles: The SentiNot Study. Ann Surg Oncol. 2023; https://doi.org/10.1245/s10434-022-13064-0. Epub ahead of print.
52. Omoto K, et al. Sentinel node detection in breast cancer using contrast-enhanced sonography with 25% albumin--initial clinical experience. J Clin Ultrasound. 2006;34:317–26.

53. Li J, et al. How pre-operative sentinel lymph node contrast-enhanced ultrasound helps intra-operative sentinel lymph node biopsy in breast cancer: initial experience. Ultrasound Med Biol. 2019;45:1865–73.
54. Sever AR, et al. Preoperative localization of sentinel lymph nodes using intradermal microbubbles and contrast-enhanced ultrasonography in patients with breast cancer. Br J Surg. 2009;96:1295–9.
55. Omoto K, et al. Sentinel node detection method using contrast-enhanced ultrasonography with sonazoid in breast cancer: preliminary clinical study. Ultrasound Med Biol. 2009;35:1249–56.
56. Sever AR, et al. Preoperative sentinel node identification with ultrasound using microbubbles in patients with breast cancer. AJR Am J Roentgenol. 2011;196:251–6.
57. Sever AR, et al. Preoperative needle biopsy of sentinel lymph nodes using intradermal microbubbles and contrast-enhanced ultrasound in patients with breast cancer. AJR Am J Roentgenol. 2012;199:465–70.
58. Hu H, Wei W, Sun D, Liu Y. [Clinical application of sentinel lymph node biopsy under the guidance of contrast-enhanced ultrasound plus methylene blue in patients with breast cancer]. Zhonghua Yi Xue Za Zhi. 2013;93:1255–7.
59. Barentsz MW, et al. Sentinel lymph node localization with contrast-enhanced ultrasound and an I-125 seed: an ideal prospective development study. Int J Surg Lond. 2015;14:1–6.
60. Matsuzawa F, et al. Accurate diagnosis of axillary lymph node metastasis using contrast-enhanced ultrasonography with Sonazoid. Mol Clin Oncol. 2015;3:299–302.
61. Xie F, et al. Intradermal microbubbles and contrast-enhanced ultrasound (CEUS) is a feasible approach for sentinel lymph node identification in early-stage breast cancer. World J Surg Oncol. 2015;13:319.
62. Eshefani, et al. Validation of contrast enhanced ultrasound technique to wire localization of sentinel lymph node in patients with early breast cancer. Indian J Surg Oncol. 2015;6. https://pubmed-ncbi-nlm-nih-gov.ezproxy.its.uu.se/27065663/?utm_source=gquery&utm_medium=referral&utm_campaign=CitationSensor.
63. Rautiainen S, et al. Contrast-enhanced ultrasound -guided axillary lymph node core biopsy: diagnostic accuracy in preoperative staging of invasive breast cancer. Eur J Radiol. 2015;84:2130–6.
64. Britton P, et al. Microbubble detection and ultrasound-guided vacuum-assisted biopsy of axillary lymph nodes in patients with breast cancer. Clin Radiol. 2017;72:772–9.
65. Shimazu K, et al. Identification of sentinel lymph nodes by contrast-enhanced ultrasonography with Sonazoid in patients with breast cancer: a feasibility study in three hospitals. Cancer Med. 2017;6:1915–22.
66. Wang Y, et al. Variation of sentinel lymphatic channels (SLCs) and sentinel lymph nodes (SLNs) assessed by contrast-enhanced ultrasound (CEUS) in breast cancer patients. World J Surg Oncol. 2017;15:127.
67. Cox K, et al. Enhanced pre-operative axillary staging using intradermal microbubbles and contrast-enhanced ultrasound to detect and biopsy sentinel lymph nodes in breast cancer: a potential replacement for axillary surgery. Br J Radiol. 2018;91:20170626.
68. Zhao J, et al. The value of contrast-enhanced ultrasound for sentinel lymph node identification and characterisation in pre-operative breast cancer patients: a prospective study. Eur Radiol. 2018;28:1654–61.
69. Zhong J, et al. Contrast-enhanced ultrasound-guided fine-needle aspiration for sentinel lymph node biopsy in early-stage breast cancer. Ultrasound Med Biol. 2018;44:1371–8.
70. Liu J, et al. Percutaneous contrast-enhanced ultrasound for localization and diagnosis of sentinel lymph node in early breast cancer. Sci Rep. 2019;9:13545.
71. Dellaportas D, et al. Contrast-enhanced color Doppler ultrasonography for preoperative evaluation of sentinel lymph node in breast cancer patients. Breast Care. 2015;10:331–5.
72. Saidha NK, Aggarwal R, Sen A. Identification of sentinel lymph nodes using contrast-enhanced ultrasound in breast cancer. Indian J Surg Oncol. 2018;9:355–61.
73. Mok CW, Tan S-M, Zheng Q, Shi L. Network meta-analysis of novel and conventional sentinel lymph node biopsy techniques in breast cancer. BJS Open. 2019;3:445–52.

74. Goyal A. New technologies for Sentinel lymph node detection. Breast Care. 2018;13:349–53.
75. Motomura K, Izumi T, Tateishi S, Tamaki Y, Ito Y, Horinouchi T, Nakanishi K. Superparamagnetic iron oxide-enhanced MRI at 3T for accurate axillary staging in breast cancer. Br J Surg. 2016;103(1):60–9.
76. Jazrawi A, Pantiora E, Abdsaleh S, et al. Magnetic-Guided Axillary UltraSound (MagUS) Sentinel lymph node biopsy and mapping in patients with early breast cancer. a phase 2, single-arm prospective clinical trial. Cancers (Basel). 2021;13(17):4285. https://doi.org/10.3390/cancers13174285. Published 2021 Aug 25.

Indocyanine Green (ICG) Dye: An Essential Element in the Breast Cancer Management Tool Kit

9

Chaitanyanand B. Koppiker, Madhura Kulkarni, Devaki A. Kelkar, and Sneha Joshi

9.1 What Is Indocyanine Green (ICG)

Indocyanine green (ICG) is one of the fluorophore probes with near-infrared light (NIR) spectra of 700–850 nm that has gained vast interest in several medical applications due to its minimal interfering absorption, inexpensive excitation and enhanced diffusion in the lymphovascular system [1].

It is a water-soluble, anionic, tricarbocyanine dye (Fig. 9.1a), showing binding affinity towards plasma and lymph globulins, especially albumin and some lipoproteins. It spreads rapidly and uniformly in the lymphatic system due to its low molecular weight and, after dermal injection, shows 98% binding to serum/lymphatic globulins [2]. The ICG dye binds to the plasma lymph proteins without altering the protein structure [3] and is exclusively cleared from circulation via the liver, where its transport is done by the bile protein glutathione *S*-transferase [2]. It also shows no toxicity or hypersensitivity when injected in human subjects.

ICG fluorophore has absorption maximum in the human circulatory system at around 800 nm (Fig. 9.1b), at which tissue absorption is at minimum. Hence, ICG gives sharp contrast for selective identification of injected tissue with minimal

C. B. Koppiker (✉)
Orchids Breast Health Centre, Pune, Maharashtra, India

Prashanti Cancer Care Mission (PCCM), Pune, Maharashtra, India

Center for Translational Cancer Research, a Joint Initiative Between IISER Pune and PCCM Pune, Pune, India
e-mail: dr.koppiker@prashanticancercare.org

M. Kulkarni · D. A. Kelkar · S. Joshi
Prashanti Cancer Care Mission (PCCM), Pune, Maharashtra, India

Center for Translational Cancer Research, a Joint Initiative Between IISER Pune and PCCM Pune, Pune, India
e-mail: madhura.kulkarni@prashanticancercare.org; dakelkar@prashanticancercare.org; snehajoshi@prashanticancercare.org

Chintamani (ed.), *Sentinel Node Biopsy in Breast Cancer*,
https://doi.org/10.1007/978-81-322-3994-9_9

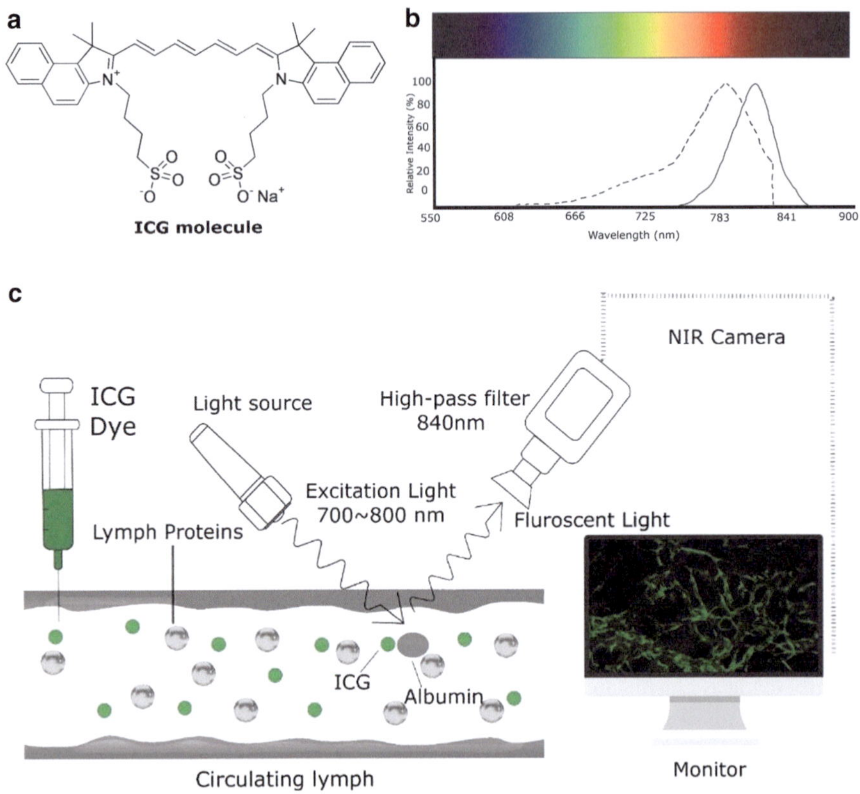

Fig. 9.1 ICG chemical structure and fluorescence spectrum: (**a**) chemical structure of Indocyanine green. (**b**) Excitation and emission spectrum of ICG in the near infrared region. The excitation peak at low dilution is at ~800 nm with an emission peak at ~830 nm. (**c**) When injected into tissue, ICG rapidly binds to proteins in the lymph. ICG is excited by an infrared source, and emission is recorded by a camera at ~840 nm to visualise lymphatic pathways in the tissue

background fluorescence. The fluorophore works in what is referred to as a tissue optical window. As seen in Fig. 9.1c, the NIR light used both in ICG excitation and fluorescence emission of ICG pierces the tissue several millimetres. This helps to observe even the lymphatic/vascular structures that might be buried deep in the tissue [4]. Intra-operative, real-time visualisation of the ICG fluorescence is done using a colour-and-fluorescence-merged imaging system (ICFIS), which aids the identification of even subcutaneous lymph vessels [5].

9.2 Dual Role for ICG Dye in Breast Cancer Management

ICG dye was first introduced in the medical setting to test for liver and cardiac dysfunction in 1959 after FDA approval [6]. ICG was introduced for sentinel lymph node visualisation in breast cancers in the year 1999 by Motomura et al. [7]. With the introduction of the charge-coupled devices, Kitai et al. for the first time in 2005 used ICG as a NIR fluorophore rather than just a dye in their cohort of 18 Breast Cancer patients [8]. The study used both clinical observation of ICG dye passage after areolar injection visually and fluorescent imaging by a charged-coupled Device (CCD) camera. The node identification rate by fluorescent imaging was found to be superior to visual observation of the green dye. Subsequently, several studies compared sentinel node identification by ICG to the standard-of-care procedure with dual-dye technique that uses radioactive colloid and blue dye for sentinel node identification, proving it to be a comparable sentinel lymph node (SLN) identification method [9–11]. The advantages of using ICG over other methods in SLN identification in both early-stage breast cancers and in neo-adjuvant settings are appreciated since then, which will be discussed here. Oncoplastic surgery today is being widely used as the standard of care in breast cancer. ICG dye is used for vascular assessment to improve the safety of oncoplastic breast surgery (OBS). The second role of ICG dye is evident in OBS. One is able to ascertain the vascularity and take steps intra-operatively to prevent flap necrosis, fat necrosis and complications in post-OBS situations by using ICG to assess vascularity in mastectomy flaps in the skin and nipple-sparing mastectomy as well as vascularity of local and remote flaps for reconstruction such as perforator flaps. This use of ICG in oncoplastic surgery opens out new advantages, which will be discussed later in the chapter.

9.3 Role of ICG in Sentinel Node Identification

Accurate SLN identification has positively impacted precision breast cancer management while reducing morbidity. The sentinel node is the first and/or closest node to the tumour that receives lymphatic drainage. Once the dye concentrates in the albumin-rich sentinel nodes, there is a lag of around 15–20 min before which it diffuses into other nodes. In the neoadjuvant chemotherapy (NACT), setting too, accurate SLN identification predicts axillary involvement and hence finds its place even in patients presenting with cN1 disease. Sentinel node procedures have become standard of care in both de novo and post NACT settings, sparing axillary lymph node (ALN)-associated morbidity (NSABP B-32 trial) [12] (Fig. 9.2).

Methylene blue dye was the first dye employed to identify SLN in breast cancer [13, 14]. On peri-tumoural injection, the dye diffuses into the sentinels, which are the closest nodes to the tumour, and these can be easily picked up for pathological assessment. By 1995, radioisotope technetium-99m (Tc)-labelled nanocolloid was introduced for SLN identification [15], where radioisotope is injected in the peri-tumoural region, and 'hot' sentinel nodes are identified using a scintillation counter. After a steep learning curve in optimising the SLN identification with both the dyes, identification rates of up to 90% were achieved with either blue dye or radioisotope alone. Later, multiple trials proved dual-modality techniques to be superior in SLN identification with identification rates of up to 96% [16, 17], advocating it as a standard of care.

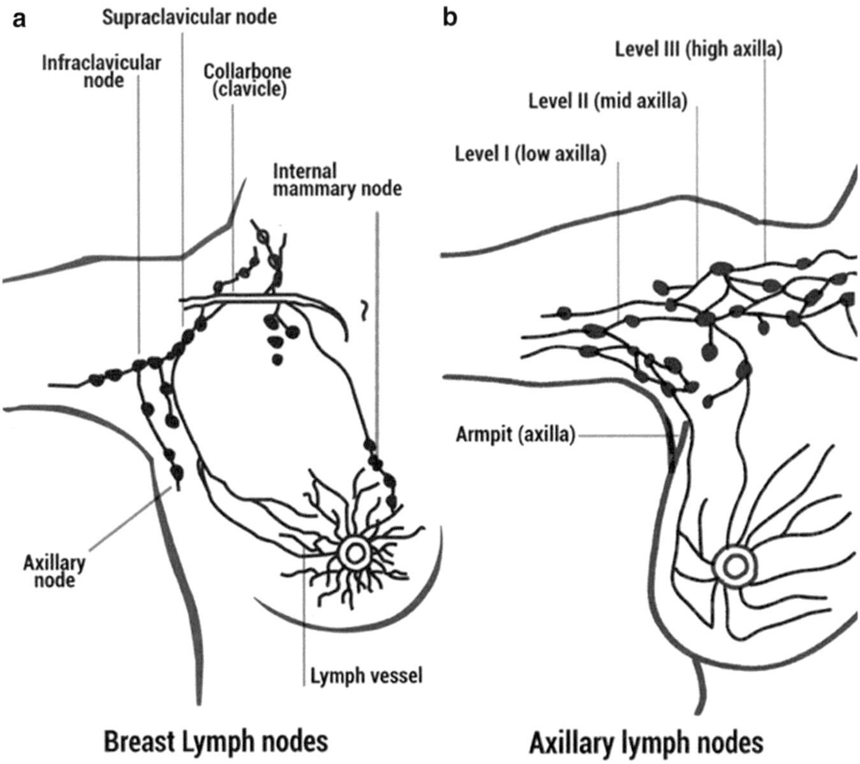

Fig. 9.2 Depiction of the anatomical location of the axillary lymphatic system. (**a**) The axillary lymphatic system extends from the axilla to the clavicular nodes and internal mammary nodes. (**b**) The axillary nodes can be classified as Levels I–III defined by the pectoralis minor muscle. Level I nodes are below the edge, Level II nodes are under and Level III nodes are above the muscle

Though the dual-dye technique increased the identification rates substantially, the radioisotope is expensive, needs licensing and carries the risk of exposure to radiation; furthermore, when using radioisotopes, there are difficulties in availing the radioactive tracer, especially in low-resource settings and developing countries [18, 19]. Various alternative techniques such as superparamagnetic iron oxide (SPIO), contrast-enhanced ultrasound scan (CEUS), ICG and fluorescein have been tested to replace the radioisotope technique [20]. SPIO replaces the radioactive substance with magnetic particles, where a special hand-held magnetometer probe is used for detection. The identification rates with SPIO are seen to drop with subcutaneous detection, and the browning of the skin tends to last longer, up to 1 year, making it a less favourable choice [21]. Under the guidance of ultrasonography, contrast-enhancing tracers like SonoVue and Sonazoid are used to localise SLN with the CEUS technique (Sever et al. [22]; Omoto et al. 23). The meta-analysis comparing the identification rates between CEUS and dual-tracer technique showed variable results for CEUS, with the need for a larger prospective trial [24]. Fluorescein is the newest dye introduced, which is in the visible range and does not need any specific equipment for visualisation, making it a promising choice. Fluorescein is adopted for retinal angiography but could not hold the promise in comparison with ICG for SLN identification due to vascular leakage and low visibility of deeper-lying blood vessels [25]. Also, it has been documented that in ophthalmic angiography, the side effects of fluorescein are greater than those of ICG [26, 27] In addition, the long half-life of fluorescein (~12 h) compared with 3–5 min for ICG makes it difficult to administer repeated injections of the dye that may be required for the surgical procedure [28].

Thus, ICG stands comparable with radioisotope with identification rates in the range of 94–100% in a dual-modality setting with blue dye and better than blue dye [9–11, 18, 19, 29].

9.4 ICG Procedure for SLNB Identification

With the standard dose of less than 2 mg/kg, ICG is a non-toxic dye with minimal side effects during intra-operative surgery, with very good reproducibility [30]. ICG provides an accurate mapping of draining lymph nodes for optimal staging and resection. The dose concentration of ICG and injection volume for optimal imaging has evolved through the years [20]. As the fluorescence capture devices have become more sensitive, smaller concentration with high-contrast cameras performs well for accurate lymph node mapping with excellent reproducibility. In our setting, 25 mg of ICG is diluted in 10-ml sterile water with a final concentration of 2.5 mg/ml, of which 0.05-ml solution is injected intradermally in the peri-areolar region at two locations (Fig. 9.3). It is the surgeon's choice whether to go for a peri-tumoural or peri-areolar injection. In our experience, with peri-areolar injection, the dye is picked up by the lymphatic plexus near the areola and is quickly transmitted to the axilla. When the tumour lies closer to the axilla, with the possibility of blocking the lymphatics, the surgeon may give an extra injection in the skin over the tumour. The volume of the injection is one of the factors that need to be considered to choose between these two options, along with the time taken between injection and the removal of SLN, where a longer time (15–20 min) may lead to diffusion. The breast may be massaged to aid the dispersal of the dye, and within 5–7 min, the sentinel node with the fluorescence dye is visualised using a hand-held multispectral camera with infrared light at 805 nm (Fig. 9.3). The SLNs are resected and assessed by frozen section examination. In breast cancer SLN mapping, ICG along with blue dye (dual modality) is used in both early-stage disease and post-NACT settings with excellent identification rates.

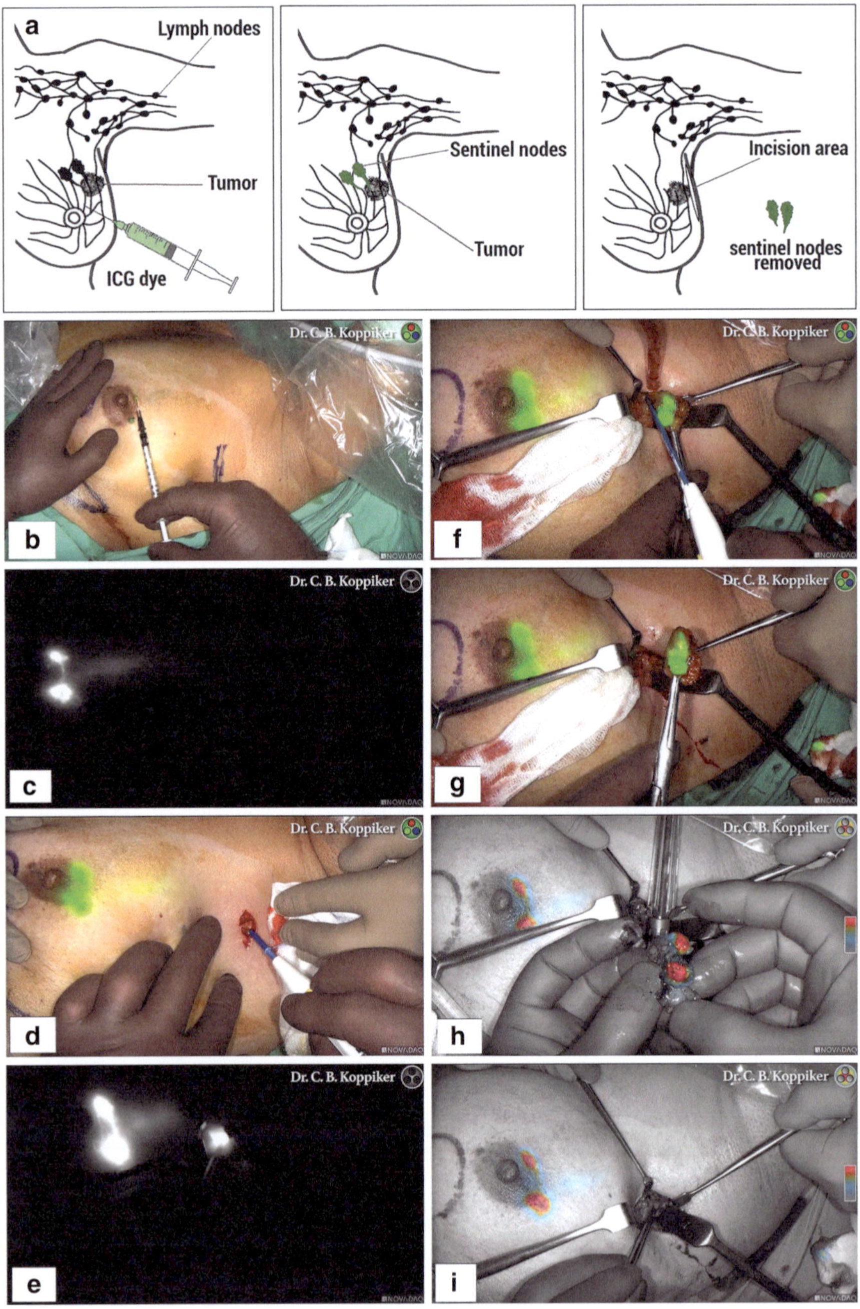
a
Lymph nodes
Tumor
ICG dye
Sentinel nodes
Tumor
Incision area
sentinel nodes removed
b
c
d
e
f
g
h
i
Dr. C. B. Koppiker

Fig. 9.3 ICG-guided sentinel lymph node biopsy: A schematic of ICG-guided SNLB. (**a**) ICG is injected in the peri-areolar region. ICG travels through the lymphatic channels, and the first nodes that fluoresce are the sentinel nodes. Guided by a fluorescent camera the nodes are dissected out. (**b–i**) ICG-guided SNLB in a breast-conserving surgery. (**b**) ICG is injected at two places in the peri-areolar region (**c**). The spy mode of the camera shows the injection points and ICG illuminating the lymphatic channels to the sentinel node. (**d**) The sentinel node (green in the colour-segmented fluorescence mode) is then identified and accessed through a new incision. (**e–h**) Two ICG-positive nodes are dissected out and can be visualised in colour-segmented fluorescence mode, overlay fluorescence mode and spy contrast mode. (**i**) In post sentinel node dissection, no further ICG is detected in the cavity (seen in overlay mode)

9.5 ICG for SLN Identification in Early-Stage Breast Cancer

Loco-regional metastasis of breast cancer occurs primarily through the lymphatic system. To achieve loco-regional control of the disease and to guide adjuvant therapy, the most important knowledge is of the lymph node status. The lymph node status further helps stage and prognosticate the disease.

SLN biopsy is the current standard of care for axillary lymphatic status in node-negative early-stage breast cancers. The conventional axillary dissection is associated with lymphedema, pain, shoulder stiffness, seroma formation, vascular injuries, swelling of the arm, sensory loss and other complications [16].

Literature supports the fact that ICG is an acceptable alternative method for SLNB. A 2015 meta-analysis by Ahmed et al. [9] demonstrated that ICG was superior to blue dye (BD) as regards the identification rate of SLNs. In 2016 Zhang et al. pooled 19 studies involving 2594 patients to show that ICG fluorescence-guided SLNB in breast cancer has a 98% detection rate for sentinel nodes. The false-negative rate was fairly low. In the presence of metastases, the method showed relatively high sensitivity and specificity as compared with a combination of BD and RI. [11].

Sugie et al. then reported with 12 studies, involving 1736 patients, a direct comparison of the diagnostic performance for ICG fluorescence and RI. They concluded that the ICG fluorescence method was better at determining axillary staging compared with the RI method [10]. In 2019, Mok et al. conducted a meta-analysis that included 35 cohort studies with 4244 subjects. In this analysis, they compared the ICG fluorescence technique with SPIO, Tc, dual-modality (Tc/BD) and CEUS. They observed that the ICG fluorescence technique performed the best in terms of detection and had the lowest false-negative rate as compared with other techniques [19]. The 2020 meta-analysis by Goonawardena and colleagues reported no statistically significant difference in SLN detection rates and sensitivity between ICG fluorescence and RI. They observed through their analysis that the sensitivity of dual mapping (ICG + RI) was better than ICG alone [9–11, 18, 19, 29].

A summary of various studies and meta-analyses indicated that ICG alone is a better tracer agent than BD or RI alone and is comparable with the dual-tracer system of BD and RI together. A standardised dose of ICG can increase detectability and precision. Considering the clinical convenience of ICG, it may be used as a suitable alternative to traditional tracers to detect SLNs in patients with breast cancer. Recently, ICG as a single modality for SLN mapping is being tested for its identification rates.

9.6 ICG for SLN Identification in Post-NACT Setting

In breast cancer patients with cN1 disease, detection of more than three sentinel nodes gave better identification rates and lesser false-negative rates in the post-NACT setting as shown in Sentinel Node Biopsy Following Neoadjuvant Chemotherapy (SN FNAC), Sentina and The American College of Surgeons Oncology Group (ACOSOG-Z1071) trials [31–34]. In fact, even in de novo early-stage breast cancer, it has been shown that the more nodes are removed (up to 3), the lesser the false-negative rate [19]. Better SLN identification saves ALND, reducing chances of lymphedema post-surgery without affecting survival outcomes in patients [35]. In the post-NACT setting, the conventional methods can lead to inadequate identification rates, failed mapping and tracing of less than three lymph nodes [36]. Thus, in a post-NACT setting, ICG gives an advantage with a a better pick-up rate due to better diffusion of small-molecular-weight ICG dye. A detailed investigation by a study to assess any effect of NACT on lymphatic routes and thereby SLN identification was done using ICG [37]. The authors showed using ICG that the lymphatic routes were unaffected by NACT and that ICG could be as effective in identifying SLN in a post-NACT setting [37]. Further, using ICG in dual-modality setting with radioisotope in comparison with radioisotope alone showed comparable identification rates. Contrarily, Mok et al. has shown that ICG has the highest node identification rate than other modalities [19]. This ability to detect more nodes gives ICG an advantage in the post-NACT setting, and we believe that a randomised controlled trial should be conducted to ascertain this advantage.

9.7 ICG in the Reverse Mapping of Lymphatic Drainage

In some patients, complete ALND is needed when they present with advanced disease. ALN dissection can lead to complications like lymphedema of the arm, which creates unnecessary morbidity. Preventing this lymphedema could be made possible by preserving the upper lymphatic drainage pathways using axillary reverse mapping (ARM). Such a procedure was first performed using blue dye and Radioisotopes (RI) by [38]. ICG dye was shown to have better sensitivity in locating the draining lymphatics in the ARM setting [39]. The utility of ARM in SLN mapping in breast cancer was described by Sakurai et al. [40]. ICG has been shown to be superior in comparison with current dyes in use, such as isosulfan blue [41] and methylene blue [42]. Conclusive studies are needed for the introduction of ICG as a standard of care in ARM procedures.

9.8 Tracking Lymphatic Drainage Post Breast Cancer Surgery with ICG

Changes in lymphatic drainage pathways that lead to breast and/or arm lymphedema are common long-term complications of breast cancer treatment [43]. Radiation scintigraphy for lymphatics has many of the same disadvantages as sentinel node identification by the radiocolloid tracer. Visualisation of the drainage pathways in the ipsilateral arm by ICG helps identify altered drainage pathways prior to clinical symptoms and assists the application of manual lymphatic drainage or surgical interventions [44]. Similar methods have also been used to visualise post-operative breast lymphoedema [45].

9.9 ICG in Oncoplastic Breast Surgeries

After IV injection of the ICG dye, vascularity assessments at the site of surgery can be easily done. OBS can be made safer with the reduction of post-operative complications such as flap necrosis, wound dehiscence, fat necrosis etc., with the help of intra-operative assessment of vascularity. Assessment of vascularity using ICG dye in nipple-areola sparing mastectomy flaps, as well as in perforator and remote flaps like DIEP, has significantly decreased the occurrence of complications [46, 47]. The most common method of assessing perforator integrity is by hand-held Doppler ultrasound and subjective clinical judgement of an experienced surgeon [47]. Dye-based tracking of perfusion has become possible with the use of ICG, an agent to visualise and image perfusion intra-operatively [47, 48] Flap ischemia is a major cause of skin necrosis post-reconstruction. An analysis of ICG angiography compared with clinical assessment of mastectomy skin flap vasculature in implant-based breast reconstruction showed significantly reduced severe flap necrosis in the ICG group [49]. Flap perfusion by ICG angiography is easily assessed visually but can also be evaluated quantitatively. Krishnan and colleagues evaluated fluorescence of the flap and found that maximal fluorescence is reached ~2 min after dye injection and lasts for 8–10 min [50]. Regions of the flap that do not fluoresce in this time window have reduced perfusion, which can then be corrected surgically. Another study showed that an increase of less than 25% fluorescence intensity over baseline identifies a non-viable skin flap 90% of the time, whereas flaps with ≥45% intensity have intact perforators >98% of the time [51]. At present, imaging systems provide false colour images of ICG fluorescence intensity (overlay fluorescence mode in Fig. 9.3) based on such quantitative studies that aid the surgeon to assess the perfusion levels (i.e. increased ICG fluorescence intensity in the tissue over baseline). The quality of perfusion in the prepared flap is therefore assessed and corrected if required intra-operatively, reducing post-surgical complications that may have arisen from inaccurate intra-operative clinical assessment [52]. Perfusion evaluation using ICG in an OBS is illustrated in Fig. 9.4.

ICG therefore finds a place in various aspects related to breast cancer surgery. Additionally ICG has been shown to be a reliable tracer in sentinel node

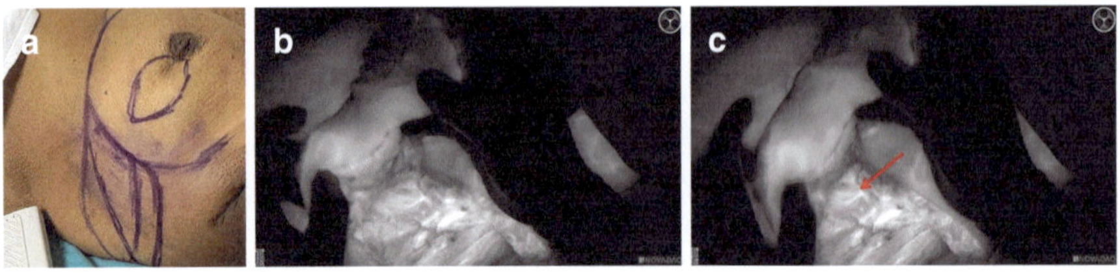

Fig. 9.4 Oncoplastic flap perfusion evaluated by ICG: images are taken from a lateral thoracic artery perforator (LTAP) flap volume replacement oncoplastic surgery. The patient received ICG intravenously. (**a**) Pre-operative markings for LTAP Flap. (**b**) Spy contrast mode image of the intact perforator. (**c**) Spy contrast mode image showing the vascularisation and the intact perforator (red arrow)

identification in other cancers such as head and neck carcinomas and melanoma [53]. Once the use of ICG and the intra-operative imaging systems have been established, it can be used for multiple conditions, making it cost-effective.

9.10 ICG as an Ideal Method for Developing Countries

The current standard of care for SLN mapping in breast cancer management uses a dual-dye technique with blue dye and radioisotope. Radioisotope needs licencing and nuclear medicine facilities in the institutions for its medical use. The radioisotope's production, transportation and disposal are tightly regulated under such licences. In low-resource settings such as India, financially sound institutions and hospitals in big cities can afford the investment in such facilities, which are a small percentage of all medical institutions in the country. Besides, the supply of radioisotope itself is unreliable due to ageing production plants and lack of maintenance thereof. As a result, the majority of centres in low-resource settings rely upon blue dye tracer that, when used as a single modality, not only has side effects such as skin necrosis but also has a very low identification rate of up to 84%.

With this backdrop, ICG proves to be an ideal candidate for dual-modality lymphatic mapping of the tumour in countries like India. It is easy to access with minimal regulatory requirements and affordable time setup cost for image capture equipment; even second- and third-tier institutions can easily afford the setup. The equipment can be shared by multiple departments in a mutispeciality hospital due to its widespread applications in GI, gynaecology, liver surgery, etc. As discussed earlier, ICG along with blue dye in a dual-modality setting gives excellent identification rates of SLN, providing the at-par standard of care similar to that of the radioisotope. With the example of our clinic, ICG can be effectively used in oncoplastic procedures by evaluating the perfusion of the flaps so as to reduce complications such as fat necrosis, flap necrosis, etc., with better surgical as well as oncological outcomes. With the strong evidence of comparable identification rates, ICG can potentially become the standard of care in breast cancer management, especially in low-resource settings.

Acknowledgments The authors would like to thank all participants who consented to participate in this chapter. We acknowledge Bajaj Auto Ltd. for providing support to research activities at Prashanti Cancer Care Mission, Pune.

We are thankful to Ms. Laleh Busheri, Ms. Smeeta Nare and Digvijay Thorat for their support in the preparation of this book chapter.

References

1. Escobedo JO, Rusin O, Lim S, Strongin RM. NIR dyes for bioimaging applications. Curr Opin Chem Biol. 2010;14(1):64–70. https://doi.org/10.1016/j.cbpa.2009.10.022.
2. Engel E, Schraml R, Maisch T, Kobuch K, König B, Szeimies R-M, Hillenkamp J, Bäumler W, Vasold R. Light-induced decomposition of indocyanine green. Invest Ophthalmol Vis Sci. 2008;49(5):1777–83. https://doi.org/10.1167/iovs.07-0911.
3. Kochubey VI, Kulyabina TV, Tuchin VV, Altshuler GB. Spectral characteristics of indocyanine green upon its interaction with biological tissues. Opt Spectrosc. 2005;99(4):560–6. https://doi.org/10.1134/1.2113369.
4. Nussbaum ES, Defillo A, Nussbaum L. The use of indocyanine green videoangiography to optimize the dural opening for intracranial parasagittal lesions. Neurosurgery. 2012;70(1 Suppl Operative):61–4. https://doi.org/10.1227/NEU.0b013e31822ecfeb.
5. Park YM, Quan YH, Kwon KH, Cho J-G, Woo J-S, Kim B-M, Lee Y-S, Jeong JM, Kim HK, Song J-J. Endoscopic sentinel lymph node biopsy using indocyanine green-neomannosyl human serum albumin. Laryngoscope. 2018;128(4):E135–40. https://doi.org/10.1002/lary.27036.
6. Alander JT, Kaartinen I, Laakso A, Pätilä T, Spillmann T, Tuchin VV, Venermo M, Välisuo P. A review of indocyanine green fluorescent imaging in surgery. Int J Biomed Imaging. 2012;2012:940585. https://doi.org/10.1155/2012/940585.
7. Motomura K, Inaji H, Komoike Y, Kasugai T, Noguchi S, Koyama H. Sentinel node biopsy guided by indocyanine green dye in breast cancer patients. Jpn J Clin Oncol. 1999;29(12):604–7. https://doi.org/10.1093/jjco/29.12.604.
8. Kitai T, Inomoto T, Miwa M, Shikayama T. Fluorescence navigation with Indocyanine green for detecting sentinel lymph nodes in breast cancer. Breast Cancer. 2005;12(3):211–5. https://doi.org/10.2325/jbcs.12.211.
9. Ahmed M, Purushotham AD, Douek M. Novel techniques for sentinel lymph node biopsy in breast cancer: a systematic review. Lancet Oncol. 2014;15(8):e351–62. https://doi.org/10.1016/S1470-2045(13)70590-4.
10. Sugie T, Kinoshita T, Masuda N, Sawada T, Yamauchi A, Kuroi K, Taguchi T, et al. Evaluation of the clinical utility of the ICG fluorescence method compared with the radioisotope method for sentinel lymph node biopsy in breast cancer. Ann Surg Oncol. 2016;23(1):44–50. https://doi.org/10.1245/s10434-015-4809-4.
11. Zhang X, Li Y, Zhou Y, Mao F, Lin Y, Guan J, Sun Q. Diagnostic performance of Indocyanine green-guided sentinel lymph node biopsy in breast cancer: a meta-analysis. PLoS One. 2016;11(6):e0155597. https://doi.org/10.1371/journal.pone.0155597.
12. Giuliano AE, Ballman KV, McCall L, Beitsch PD, Brennan MB, Kelemen PR, Ollila DW, et al. Effect of axillary dissection vs no axillary dissection on 10-year overall survival among women with invasive breast cancer and sentinel node metastasis: the ACOSOG Z0011 (Alliance) randomized clinical trial. JAMA. 2017;318(10):918–26. https://doi.org/10.1001/jama.2017.11470.
13. Giuliano AE, Jones RC, Brennan M, Statman R. Sentinel lymphadenectomy in breast cancer. J Clin Oncol. 1997;15(6):2345–50. https://doi.org/10.1200/JCO.1997.15.6.2345.
14. Giuliano AE, Kirgan DM, Guenther JM, Morton DL. Lymphatic mapping and sentinel lymphadenectomy for breast cancer. Ann Surg. 1994;220(3):391–401. https://doi.org/10.1097/00000658-199409000-00015.

15. Krag DN, Weaver DL, Alex JC, Fairbank JT. Surgical resection and radiolocalization of the sentinel lymph node in breast cancer using a gamma probe. Surg Oncol. 1993;2(6):335–9; discussion 340. https://doi.org/10.1016/0960-7404(93)90064-6.
16. Kim T, Giuliano AE, Lyman GH. Lymphatic mapping and sentinel lymph node biopsy in early-stage breast carcinoma: a Meta-analysis. Cancer. 2006;106(1):4–16. https://doi.org/10.1002/cncr.21568.
17. Pesek S, Ashikaga T, Krag LE, Krag D. The false-negative rate of sentinel node biopsy in patients with breast cancer: a meta-analysis. World J Surg. 2012;36(9):2239–51. https://doi.org/10.1007/s00268-012-1623-z.
18. Kedrzycki MS, Leiloglou M, Ashrafian H, Jiwa N, Thiruchelvam PTR, Elson DS, Leff DR. Meta-analysis comparing fluorescence imaging with radioisotope and blue dye-guided sentinel node identification for breast cancer surgery. Ann Surg Oncol. 2021;28(7):3738–48. https://doi.org/10.1245/s10434-020-09288-7.
19. Mok CW, Tan SM, Zheng Q, Shi L. Network meta-analysis of novel and conventional sentinel lymph node biopsy techniques in breast cancer. BJS Open. 2019;3(4):445–52. https://doi.org/10.1002/bjs5.50157.
20. Goyal A. New technologies for sentinel lymph node detection. Breast Care. 2018;13(5):349–53. https://doi.org/10.1159/000492436.
21. Karakatsanis A, Christiansen PM, Fischer L, Hedin C, Pistioli L, Sund M, Rasmussen NR, et al. The Nordic SentiMag trial: a comparison of super paramagnetic iron oxide (SPIO) nanoparticles versus Tc(99) and patent blue in the detection of sentinel node (SN) in patients with breast cancer and a meta-analysis of earlier studies. Breast Cancer Res Treat. 2016;157(2):281–94. https://doi.org/10.1007/s10549-016-3809-9.
22. Sever A, Jones S, Cox K, Weeks J, Mills P, Jones P. Preoperative localization of sentinel lymph nodes using intradermal microbubbles and contrast-enhanced ultrasonography in patients with breast cancer. Br J Surg. 2009;96(11):1295–9. https://doi.org/10.1002/bjs.6725. PMID: 19847869.
23. Omoto K. Futsuhara O. Sekine & M. Sakuragi. (2011). Sentinel node identification method using contrast-enhanced... https://www.umbjournal.org/article/S0301-5629(11)00714-9/fulltext.
24. Cui Q, Dai L, Li J, Xue J. Accuracy of CEUS-guided sentinel lymph node biopsy in early-stage breast cancer: a study review and meta-analysis. World J Surg Oncol. 2020;18(1):1–11. https://doi.org/10.1186/s12957-020-01890-z.
25. Freeman WR, Bartsch DU, Mueller AJ, Banker AS, Weinreb RN. Simultaneous indocyanine green and fluorescein angiography using a confocal scanning laser ophthalmoscope. Arch Ophthalmol. 1998;116(4):455–63. https://doi.org/10.1001/archopht.116.4.455.
26. Hope-Ross M, Yannuzzi LA, Gragoudas ES, Guyer DR, Slakter JS, Sorenson JA, Krupsky S, Orlock DA, Puliafito CA. Adverse reactions due to Indocyanine green. Ophthalmology. 1994;101(3):529–33. https://doi.org/10.1016/S0161-6420(94)31303-0.
27. Yannuzzi LA, Rohrer KT, Tindel LJ, Sobel RS, Costanza MA, Shields W, Zang E. Fluorescein angiography complication survey. Ophthalmology. 1986;93(5):611–7. https://doi.org/10.1016/s0161-6420(86)33697-2.
28. Gurtner GC, Jones GE, Neligan PC, Newman MI, Phillips BT, Sacks JM, Zenn MR. Intraoperative laser angiography using the SPY system: review of the literature and recommendations for use. Ann Surg Innov Res. 2013;7(1):1. https://doi.org/10.1186/1750-1164-7-1.
29. Goonawardena J, Yong C, Law M. Use of indocyanine green fluorescence compared to radioisotope for sentinel lymph node biopsy in early-stage breast cancer: systematic review and meta-analysis. Am J Surg. 2020;220(3):665–76. https://doi.org/10.1016/j.amjsurg.2020.02.001.
30. Morrell ALG, Charles MA, Morrell-Junior MAC, Mendes JM, Tustumi F, Gioia A. Indocyanine green fluorescence imaging in robotic surgery: state of art, tips and tricks in current applications. Arq Gastroenterol. 2021;58(1):61–70.
31. Boileau J-F, Poirier B, Basik M, Holloway CMB, Gaboury L, Sideris L, Meterissian S, et al. Sentinel node biopsy after neoadjuvant chemotherapy in biopsy-proven node-positive breast

cancer: the SN FNAC study. J Clin Oncol. 2015;33(3):258–64. https://doi.org/10.1200/JCO.2014.55.7827.

32. Boughey JC, Suman VJ, Mittendorf EA, Ahrendt GM, Wilke LG, Bret Taback A, Leitch M, et al. Sentinel lymph node surgery after neoadjuvant chemotherapy in patients with node-positive breast cancer: the ACOSOG Z1071 (Alliance) clinical trial. JAMA. 2013;310(14):1455–61. https://doi.org/10.1001/jama.2013.278932.
33. Classe J-M, Cecile Loaec P, Gimbergues SA, Tunon C, de Lara PF, Dupre RR, et al. Sentinel lymph node biopsy without axillary lymphadenectomy after neoadjuvant chemotherapy is accurate and safe for selected patients: the GANEA 2 study. Breast Cancer Res Treat. 2019;173(2):343–52. https://doi.org/10.1007/s10549-018-5004-7.
34. Kuehn T, Bauerfeind I, Fehm T, Fleige B, Hausschild M, Helms G, Lebeau A, Liedtke C. Sentinel-lymph-node biopsy in patients with breast cancer before and after neoadjuvant chemotherapy (SENTINA): a prospective, multicentre cohort study. Lancet Oncol. 2013;14(7):609–18. https://doi.org/10.1016/S1470-2045(13)70166-9.
35. Pilewskie M, Morrow M. Axillary nodal management following neoadjuvant chemotherapy: a review. JAMA Oncol. 2017;3(4):549–55. https://doi.org/10.1001/jamaoncol.2016.4163.
36. Mamtani A, Barrio AV, King TA, Van Zee KJ, Plitas G, Pilewskie M, El-Tamer M, et al. How often does neoadjuvant chemotherapy avoid axillary dissection in patients with histologically confirmed nodal metastases? Results of a prospective study. Ann Surg Oncol. 2016;23(11):3467–74. https://doi.org/10.1245/s10434-016-5246-8.
37. Tsuyuki S, Yamaguchi A, Senda N, Kawata Y, Kawaguchi K. Effect of neoadjuvant chemotherapy on lymphatic pathways leading to sentinel lymph nodes in breast cancer. Cancer Cell Microenviron. 2015;2. https://doi.org/10.14800/ccm.850.
38. Noguchi M, Noguchi M, Nakano Y, Ohno Y, Kosaka T. Axillary reverse mapping using a fluorescence imaging system in breast cancer. J Surg Oncol. 2012;105(3):229–34. https://doi.org/10.1002/jso.22094.
39. Ikeda K, Ogawa Y, Komatsu H, Mori Y, Ishikawa A, Nakajima T, Oohira G, Tokunaga S, Fukushima H, Inoue T. Evaluation of the metastatic status of lymph nodes identified using axillary reverse mapping in breast cancer patients. World J Surg Oncol. 2012;10:233. https://doi.org/10.1186/1477-7819-10-233.
40. Sakurai T, Endo M, Shimizu K, Yoshimizu N, Nakajima K, Nosaka K, Dai Y, Iwao A, Jinnai Y. Axillary reverse mapping using fluorescence imaging is useful for identifying the risk group of postoperative lymphedema in breast cancer patients undergoing sentinel node biopsies. J Surg Oncol. 2014;109(6):612–5. https://doi.org/10.1002/jso.23528.
41. Foster D, Choy N, Porter C, Ahmed S, Wapnir I. Axillary reverse mapping with Indocyanine green or isosulfan blue demonstrate similar crossover rates to radiotracer identified sentinel nodes. J Surg Oncol. 2018;117(3):336–40. https://doi.org/10.1002/jso.24859.
42. Wu J-D, Wang Z, Zeng H-C, He L-F, Zhang Y-Q, Huang G-S, Zhang F, Wei X-L, Huang W-H, Zhang G-J. Comparison of indocyanine green and methylene blue use for axillary reverse mapping during axillary lymph node dissection. MedComm. 2020;1(2):211–8. https://doi.org/10.1002/mco2.31.
43. Paskett ED, Dean JA, Oliveri JM, Phil J, Harrop. Cancer-related lymphedema risk factors, diagnosis, treatment, and impact: a review. J Clin Oncol. 2012;30(30):3726–33. https://doi.org/10.1200/JCO.2012.41.8574.
44. Suami H. Anatomical theories of the pathophysiology of cancer-related lymphoedema. Cancers. 2020;12(5):1338. https://doi.org/10.3390/cancers12051338.
45. Heydon-White A, Suami H, Boyages J, Koelmeyer L, Peebles KC. Assessing breast lymphoedema following breast cancer treatment using indocyanine green lymphography. Breast Cancer Res Treat. 2020;181(3):635–44. https://doi.org/10.1007/s10549-020-05661-y.
46. Anker AM, Prantl L, Strauss C, Brébant V, Schenkhoff F, Pawlik M, Vykoukal J, Klein SM. Assessment of DIEP flap perfusion with intraoperative Indocyanine green fluorescence imaging in vasopressor-dominated hemodynamic support versus Liberal fluid administration: a randomized controlled trial with breast cancer patients. Ann Surg Oncol. 2020;27(2):399–406. https://doi.org/10.1245/s10434-019-07758-1.

47. Ludolph I, Arkudas A, Schmitz M, Boos AM, Taeger CD, Rother U, Horch RE, Beier JP. Cracking the perfusion code?: laser-assisted indocyanine green angiography and combined laser Doppler spectrophotometry for intraoperative evaluation of tissue perfusion in autologous breast reconstruction with DIEP or Ms-TRAM flaps. J Plast Reconstruct Aesth Surg. 2016;69(10):1382–8. https://doi.org/10.1016/j.bjps.2016.07.014.
48. Liu DZ, Mathes DW, Zenn MR, Neligan PC. The application of indocyanine green fluorescence angiography in plastic surgery. J Reconstr Microsurg. 2011;27(6):355–63. https://doi.org/10.1055/s-0031-1281515.
49. Diep GK, Hui JYC, Marmor S, Cunningham BL, Choudry U, Portschy PR, Tuttle TM. Postmastectomy reconstruction outcomes after intraoperative evaluation with indocyanine green angiography versus clinical assessment. Ann Surg Oncol. 2016;23(12):4080–5. https://doi.org/10.1245/s10434-016-5466-y.
50. Krishnan KG, Schackert G, Steinmeier R. The role of near-infrared angiography in the assessment of post-operative venous congestion in random pattern, pedicled Island and free flaps. Br J Plast Surg. 2005;58(3):330–8. https://doi.org/10.1016/j.bjps.2004.10.003.
51. Moyer HR, Losken A. Predicting mastectomy skin flap necrosis with Indocyanine green angiography: the gray area defined. Plast Reconstr Surg. 2012;129(5):1043–8. https://doi.org/10.1097/PRS.0b013e31824a2b02.
52. Reinhart MB, Huntington CR, Blair LJ, Todd Heniford B, Augenstein VA. Indocyanine green: historical context, current applications, and future considerations. Surg Innov. 2016;23(2):166–75. https://doi.org/10.1177/1553350615604053.
53. Knackstedt R, Couto RA, Ko J, Cakmakoglu C, Daisy W, Gastman B. Indocyanine green fluorescence imaging with lymphoscintigraphy for sentinel node biopsy in melanoma: increasing the sentinel lymph node-positive rate. Ann Surg Oncol. 2019;26(11):3550–60. https://doi.org/10.1245/s10434-019-07617-z.

10 Sentinel Lymph Node Biopsy (SLNB) Post-NACT and Targeted Axillary Dissection (TAD)

Urvashi Jain and Ashutosh Kothari

10.1 Introduction

Management of the axilla has seen a significant evolution over the last four decades with an increasing trend towards de-escalation to reduce morbidity and enhance quality of life (QOL) without comprising long-term oncological outcomes in breast cancer patients. The introduction of newer systemic treatments has, to a great deal, driven this approach of de-escalation. Axillary lymph node dissection (ALND) remained the standard of care for several decades until the late twentieth century. In 1971, the NSABP-B04 trial laid the foundation for de-escalation of axillary surgery. It reported no benefit in overall survival (OS) with ALND when compared with total mastectomy alone or total mastectomy followed by chest wall and regional nodal irradiation (RNI) in clinically node-negative patients with early-stage breast cancer (EBC) [1]. However, despite these results, ALND continued to be the standard of care for several years. This was primarily the case as ALND did not only provide local control but also prognostic information by accurately staging the axilla which in turn guided the recommendations for optimal adjuvant therapy. Towards the end of the twentieth century, the NSABP-B32 and a trial conducted in Milan showed that SLNB could be safely used instead of ALND to provide the same information with considerably less morbidity in patients with EBC [2, 3]. The earlier part of the twenty-first century then saw the role of ALND diminish in patients with EBC having positive sentinel nodes (SN) with trials such as AMAROS and ACOSOG-Z11 [4, 5]. This chapter will mainly focus on the potential role of diminishing ALND in patients receiving neo-adjuvant chemotherapy (NACT) based on recent evidence

U. Jain (✉)
Department of Breast Surgery, Guy's & St Thomas' NHS Foundation Trust, London, UK

A. Kothari
Department of Breast Surgery, Guy's & St Thomas' NHS Foundation Trust, London, UK

King's College, London, UK

Chintamani (ed.), *Sentinel Node Biopsy in Breast Cancer*,
https://doi.org/10.1007/978-81-322-3994-9_10

and guidelines. This concept currently applies to patients with operable breast cancer (cT1–3, N0-cN1) as the feasibility and accuracy of SLNB post-NACT are questionable in patients with locally advanced breast cancer (LABC-T4, cN2, inflammatory breast cancer).

10.2 Role of NACT in De-escalation

NACT is known to not only downstage the disease in the breast but also in the axilla.

Early randomised controlled trials (RCTs) such as the NSABP-B18, EORTC, ECTO and preliminary results of NSABP-B27 comparing NACT with primary surgery reported that NACT downstaged the axilla in 30–40% of patients receiving anthracycline- and taxane-based chemotherapy [6–9]. The advent of newer systemic and targeted therapies, especially for triple-negative breast cancer (TNBC) and Her2-positive disease, saw the pathological complete response (pCR) rates rise exponentially from approximately 20–30% to about 60% in recent trials [10–12]. NACT has given us the opportunity to downstage the axilla and minimise surgical intervention, consequently reducing the post-surgical morbidity. NACT also helps in identifying the in vivo response of tumours to systemic therapies. The post-NACT residual disease burden helps guide recommendations for additional systemic treatments [13, 14].

10.3 Sequence of SLNB and NACT

The timing of SLNB (pre-NACT SLNB vs post-NACT SLNB) has been extensively debated over the years [15, 16]. The main advantage of performing the SLNB upfront is getting to know the true pathological status of the treatment-naïve axilla, which may have therapeutic implications, particularly in the planning of adjuvant RT.

However, there are several arguments in favour of performing SLNB post-NACT. Apart from sparing the patient a separate procedure, NACT also assesses the in vivo response to systemic therapy in the axilla, and pCR is known to be a strong predictor of an improved OS. It also helps plan further treatment in certain subgroups of patients with a residual disease burden. The strongest advantage of performing SLNB post-NACT is that it converts cN0pN1 axilla to ypN0 in 20–40% of patients, thus sparing them of the additional morbidity associated with radical locoregional therapy.

10.4 Concerns with SLNB Post-NACT

There are two main concerns associated with SLNB post-NACT. One of them is regarded as the anatomical concern, where the blockage of the afferent lymphatics or then the SLNs by tumour cells or post-treatment apoptotic cells and fibrosis may divert the lymph to healthy non-SLNs, which then become the de facto SLNs. The other concern is the biological concern due to the apparent differential tumour response, wherein the tumour regression may vary in SLN versus non-SLN: the SLN may respond to the NACT, whereas non-SLNs may not respond to the NACT. Either scenario would result in decreased identification rate (IR) and increased false-negative rate (FNR). Hence, it is crucial to look at the IR and FNR when conducting trials in patients undergoing SLNB post-NACT.

10.5 Assessment of the Axilla Before NACT

The earlier trials like NSABP-B04 assessed the axilla only clinically and reported outcomes in patients with cN0 axilla. However, more recently, radiological assessment of the axilla with ultrasound and FNAC/core biopsy of the indeterminate/suspicious nodes together with a clinical assessment is considered as standard of care. This provides useful clinical information and has several advantages. It helps avoid SLNB in patients who are being planned for primary surgery. For patients being considered for NACT, this will be helpful as a tool to assess chemosensitivity by determining the response in the involved lymph node. It also helps mark the involved lymph node and localise it for future removal. Assessment of the axilla by ultrasound reports an overall sensitivity rate of 47–90% and specificity of 100% [17–19]. Sensitivity is reported to drop to 44% when the metastases in the LN is less than 5 mm but increases to 93% if the metastases is more than 5 mm in the LN, which is re-assuring to not miss clinically significant disease in the axilla [17].

10.6 Role of SLNB in cN0 Axilla Receiving NACT

The role of SLNB, as an axillary staging procedure following systematic therapy, was debated for several years due to the fear of low IR, high FNR and eventually higher loco-regional failure rates. However, data from several studies now support the use of SLNB, making it the standard of care after NACT in patients with cN0 axilla.

The largest of these published trials is NSABP B-27 [20]. This trial randomised 428 patients with clinically node-negative axilla receiving NACT to SLNB post-NACT or SLNB followed by completion ALND. They reported an IR of 85% and FNR of 11% for SLNB. A meta-analysis of 24 studies involving 1799 patients who underwent SLNB with subsequent ALND after NACT revealed an IR of 89.6% and FNR of 8.4% for SLNB [21]. Recent meta-analysis and systematic review conducted in 2016 have shown the technical feasibility and accuracy of SLNB as an acceptable axillary staging procedure in patients with initially clinically node-negative breast cancer after NACT [22]. This meta-analysis included 16 studies involving 1456 patients and reported a pooled IR of 96% and pooled FNR of 6% for SLNB, which is even lower than that in patients who underwent upfront SLNB in EBC trials without NACT. Additionally, long-term follow up data show that SLNB after systemic therapy does not lead to higher loco-regional failure rates [23].

It is important to understand the clinical relevance of these cN0 patients who are candidates for NACT as they are known to have a high rate of subclinical involvement of the axilla. In NSABP B-18, of the patients who were clinically node negative and underwent surgery first, 48% had involvement of the nodes in the axilla during surgery as compared with 33% post-NACT [6]. This rate was similar in the NSABP B-04 trial showing involvement of the axilla in about 40% of patients who were deemed cN0 by the surgeons on palpation [1]. These numbers are much lower today as the axilla is not only assessed clinically but also radiologically. Nevertheless, it also drives the point that when SLNB is done upfront, there is a possibility of finding increased subclinical axillary involvement of the axilla, and therefore, SLNB should be performed post-NACT in these cN0 patients.

10.7 Role of SLNB in cN+ Axilla Receiving NACT

After establishing the safety of SLNB in patients with cN0 axilla post-NACT, investigators started looking at the role of SLNB in patients with clinically and pathologically involved axillary LNs prior to NACT. They wanted to spare patients with an axillary complete pathological response the morbidity associated with an ALND. There have been four prospective studies that have looked at the feasibility of performing SLNB in the post-NACT setting for patients with pathological involvement of the axilla prior to NACT as shown in Table 10.1 [24–27]. In all the four studies, patients with a pathologically proven node-positive axilla who received NACT were subjected to SLNB post-NACT followed by ALND irrespective of nodal status post-NACT. As shown in Table 10.1, the overall FNR was above 10% for all the studies except SN FNAC, which reported an overall FNR of 8.4%. This

Table 10.1 Prospective trials of SLNB post-NACT in patients with biopsy-proven positive axilla prior to NACT

Trials	Sample size	SLN technique	IHC use	pCR in nodes	IR	FNR-overall	FNR-1 SLN	FNR-2 SLN	FNR-≥3 SLN
ACOSOG Z1071-USA [24]	649	Dual	No	41%	92.7%	12.9%	31.5%	21.1%	9.1%
SENTINA-Arm C-Germany [25]	692	Radio colloid	No	52%	80.1%	14.2%	24.3%	18.5%	7.3%
SN FNAC-Canada [26]	153	Radio colloid	Yes	35%	87.6%	8.4%	18.2%	4.9%	–
GANEA-2 France [27]	307	Dual	No	34%	79.5%	11.9%	19.3%	–	7.8%

can be attributed to the fact that IHC was used for nodal assessment in this study as opposed to only H&E in other studies. The use of the dual-tracer method and the number of nodes retrieved also resulted in a decrease in the FNR. The FNR significantly dropped when three or more SLNs were retrieved as compared with one SLN. However, this is not a phenomenon that occurs only in patients receiving NACT. The NSABP-B32 also demonstrated a similar trend with the SLN yield when SLN was done upfront without prior NACT [2].

A recent meta-analysis conducted in 2016, comprising of 19 studies involving 3398 patients undergoing SLNB post-NACT with pathologically proven axillary nodes prior to NACT, reported a pooled IR of 91% and pooled FNR of 13% [28]. It concluded that SLNB after NACT in biopsy-proven positive patients results in a reasonably acceptable FNR and IR, making it a valid alternative to SLNB. However, more refined patient selection and optimal techniques can improve the FNR and IR in this patient population.

10.8 Retrieval of the Clipped/Marked Node Post-NACT in Pre-NACT Node-Positive Patients

As discussed earlier, given the anatomical concerns associated with SLNB post-NACT, attempts were made to refine the techniques to decrease the FNR and establish an oncologically safe technique. Besides using the dual-tracer method and retrieving >2 SLN, a new concept of retrieving the biopsy-proven positive node was explored. A clip/marker was inserted into the biopsied node prior to starting NACT, and it was suggested that retrieving the clipped/marked node post-NACT would decrease the FNR. One of the very first observations made regarding the role of clipped node (biopsy proven to be positive prior to NACT) retrieval was in an unplanned subgroup analysis of the ACOSOG-Z1071 trial [24]. The FNR was reported to be 6.8% when the clip was retrieved in the SLNB ($n = 107$). The FNR was 19% when the clip was not identified in the SLNB ($n = 34$) but in the ALND and 13.4–14.3% if no clip was placed or if the clip was not identified ($n = 29$). The MD Anderson Cancer Centre then published their results of removal of the clipped node versus doing SLNB alone versus retrieving both the clipped node along with the SLN in all patients with node-positive breast cancer receiving NACT [29]. They reported an FNR of 10.1% when only SLNB was performed. The FNR dropped to 4.2% when only the clipped node was removed and even further down to 1.4% when SLNB was performed along with removal of the clipped node. Their results revealed that the clipped node was not the SLN in 23% of the patients, and this led to the inception of the concept of targeted axillary dissection (TAD).

M Donker et al. published their experience from Netherlands with the MARI (marking the axillary lymph nodes with radioactive iodine seeds) procedure for axillary staging after NACT in breast cancer patients [30]. They reported an IR of 97%, FNR of 7% and negative predictive value of 83.3% with this technique.

10.9 Targeted Axillary Dissection (TAD)

TAD is an axillary staging procedure performed following NACT, and it involves the removal of the marked node along with a dual-tracer SLNB in patients with proven axillary nodal involvement prior to NACT. The concept of TAD emerged to offer axillary conservation to a specific subgroup of patients (discussed above), thereby decreasing the morbidity of a radical procedure without compromising oncological outcomes. There have been several studies that have shown TAD to be a safe and accurate method of axillary staging in a certain select group of patients with documented evidence of axillary nodal involvement prior to NACT. The investigators of the RISAS (Radioactive Iodine Seed Placement in the Axilla with Sentinel Lymph Node Biopsy After Neo-Adjuvant Chemotherapy in Breast Cancer) trial, a multicentre prospective study, presented their results at the San Antonio Breast Cancer Conference (SABCS) in 2020 [31]. They enrolled 227 patients who underwent the RISAS procedure. About 35.4% (n = 79) of patients achieved pCR. They focused on the group with residual axillary disease (n = 144). Although the primary aim was to prove non-inferiority to ALND, which could not be achieved, the overall FNR was 3.47%, which was reassuringly low.

A systematic review and pooled analysis in 2021 published results of nine studies (n = 366) with marked lymph node biopsy (MLNB) and 13 studies (n = 521) with TAD [32]. It reported an overall FNR of 6.28% for MLNB alone and 5.16% for TAD. The FNRs for both the procedures were relatively lower than the FNR of 13% for SLNB alone in the same setting. The FNRs reported in this meta-analysis are also much lower than the accepted FNR of 10% (10% taken as an arbitrary cut-off in most clinical trials) for SLNB in cN0 patients, thus establishing TAD to be a viable and safe option for axillary staging in this subgroup of patients. There are several techniques used to mark and localise the initial positive lymph node before NACT for TAD which are covered in the next chapter.

10.10 Axillary Recurrence Rate for SLNB Post-NACT

It is crucial to ensure that any attempt to de-escalate axillary surgery does not worsen the oncological outcomes in patients undergoing SLNB post-NACT. Table 10.2 shows several studies that have reported axillary recurrences in these patients. The axillary recurrences are well below 2%, in fact close to 0% in majority of the studies. Although a longer follow up is required for robust evidence, these numbers are promising. Most of these studies have also shown that SLNB in these patients did not have an impact on disease-free survival (DFS) or OS when compared with ALND.

Table 10.2 Axillary recurrences in patients who underwent SLNB post-NACT

Studies	Year	Sample size	cN status prior to NACT	Median F/U (years)	Axillary recurrence (%)
Galimberti et al. [33]	2016	396	cN0–2	5	0.7%
Nogi et al. [34]	2017	183	cN0	4.3	0%
Classe et al. (GANEA-2) [27]	2019	419	cN0	3	0.2%
Kahler-Riberio-Fontana et al. [35]	2020	305	cN0	9.2	2.3%
		123	cN1–2		1.6%
Martelli et al. [36]	2020	95	cN0	9	0%
		81	cN1		0%
Piltin et al. [37]	2020	159	cN1–3	2.8	0.6%
Wong et al. [38]	2021	101	cN0	3	1%
		58	cN1–2		0%

10.11 Positive SLNB Post-NACT

Completion ALND still remains the standard of care for patients who are found to have residual disease in the SLN post-NACT outside of a clinical trial, given the risk of further disease in the remaining axilla. A study from Memorial Sloan Kettering Cancer Centre (MSKCC) in New York reported their experience of 171 patients with a positive SLNB post-NACT who underwent completion ALND [39]. The aim of the study was to identify residual burden of disease in the rest of the axilla and ascertain whether an ALND was still indicated for low-volume disease in the SLNs post-NACT. About 73% of patients in the study had documented pathologically proven node-positive disease before NACT. On completion ALND, they found one or more additional positive nodes in 17% of patients with isolated tumour cells (ITCs, 1/6), in 64% patients with micro-metastases (28/44) and in 62% patients with macro-metastases (75/121). They concluded that low-volume SLN disease after NACT is not an indicator of low risk of additional positive axillary nodes and remains an indicator of ALND outside of a clinical trial.

10.12 Future Perspectives

The quest for omission of radical surgeries to reduce morbidity continues with future trials focusing on de-escalation of the axilla in SLNB positive patients post-NACT. The British ATNEC trial is a prospective multicentre randomised trial that is currently accruing patients with T1–2, N1 disease undergoing BCS or mastectomy with TAD post-NACT with removal of at least three nodes. The patients with 1–2 positive nodes on SLNB will be randomised to either RT or ALND. The patients that are ypN0 will be randomised to either RT or ALND in one arm and no further regional treatment in the other arm with a primary endpoint of DFS at 5 years. The Alliance A011202 trial will evaluate patients with cN+ disease that convert to yN0 post-NACT and are found to have positive SLN, randomising them to ALND plus regional nodal RT (no RT to axilla) or axillary and regional nodal RT. The NEO NOD 2 is an Italian trial evaluating omission of ALND in patients with micro-metastases in post-NACT SLNB for cN1 disease. The Swiss TAXIS trial, a prospective multicentre randomised trial, is recruiting patients with cN1 or ycN1 status and Stage 2/3 disease. They will be randomised to undergo ALND or exclusive resection of clinically apparent disease including excision of clipped nodes followed by RT to the axilla, with primary endpoint of DFS at 5 years. In light of advances in systemic treatments, enriched biological understanding, and ongoing trials exploring de-escalation of axillary surgery, the management of axilla remains an intriguing and ever-evolving field, brimming with potential for further advancements.

References

1. Fisher B, et al. Twenty-five-year follow-up of a randomized trial comparing radical mastectomy, total mastectomy, and total mastectomy followed by irradiation. N Engl J Med. 2002;347(8):567–75.
2. Krag DN, et al. Sentinel-lymph-node resection compared with conventional axillary-lymph-node dissection in clinically node-negative patients with breast cancer: overall survival findings from the NSABP B-32 randomised phase 3 trial. Lancet Oncol. 2010;11(10):927–33.
3. Veronesi U, et al. A randomized comparison of sentinel-node biopsy with routine axillary dissection in breast cancer. N Engl J Med. 2003;349:546–53.
4. Donker M, et al. Radiotherapy or surgery of the axilla after a positive sentinel node in breast cancer (EORTC 10981-22023 AMAROS): a randomised, multicentre, open-label, phase 3 non-inferiority trial. Lancet Oncol. 2014;15(12):1303–10.
5. Giuliano AE, et al. Effect of axillary dissection vs no axillary dissection on 10-year overall survival among women with invasive breast cancer and sentinel node metastasis the ACOSOG Z0011 (Alliance) randomized clinical trial. JAMA. 2017;318(10):918–26.
6. Fisher B, et al. Effect of preoperative chemotherapy on local-regional disease in women with operable breast cancer: findings from National Surgical Adjuvant Breast and Bowel Project B-18. J Clin Oncol. 1997;15(7):2483–93.
7. van Nes JG, Putter H, Julien JP, et al. Preoperative chemotherapy is safe in early breast cancer, even after 10 years of follow-up; clinical and translational results from the EORTC trial 10902. Breast Cancer Res Treat. 2009;115(1):101–13.
8. Gianni L, Baselga J, Eiermann W, Guillem Porta V, Semiglazov V, Lluch A, et al. European Cooperative Trial in Operable Breast Cancer (ECTO): improved freedom from progression (FFP) by adding paclitaxel (T) to doxorubicin (A) followed by cyclophosphamide methotrexate and fluorouracil (CMF). J Clin Oncol (Meeting Abstracts). 2005;23:513.
9. Bear HD, Anderson S, Brown A, et al. The effect on tumor response of adding sequential preoperative docetaxel to preoperative doxorubicin and cyclophosphamide: preliminary results from National Surgical Adjuvant Breast and Bowel Project Protocol B-27. J Clin Oncol. 2003;21(22):4165–74.
10. Gianni L, Pienkowski T, Im Y-H, et al. 5-Year analysis of neoadjuvant pertuzumab and trastuzumab in patients with locally advanced, inflammatory, or early-stage HER2-positive breast cancer (NeoSphere): a multicentre, open-label, phase 2 randomised trial. Lancet Oncol. 2016;17(6):791–800.
11. Nanda R, Liu MC, Yau C, Shatsky R, Pusztai L, Wallace A, et al. Effect of pembrolizumab plus neoadjuvant chemotherapy on pathologic complete response in women with early-stage breast cancer: an analysis of the ongoing phase 2 adaptively randomized I-SPY2 trial. JAMA Oncol. 2020;6:676–84.

12. Mittendorf EA, Zhang H, Barrios CH, Saji S, Jung KH, Hegg R, et al. Neoadjuvant atezolizumab in combination with sequential nab-paclitaxel and anthracycline based chemotherapy versus placebo and chemotherapy in patients with early-stage triple-negative breast cancer (IMpassion031): a randomised, double-blind, phase 3 trial. Lancet. 2020;396:1090–100.
13. Masuda N, Lee SJ, Ohtani S, et al. Adjuvant capecitabine for breast cancer after preoperative chemotherapy. N Engl J Med. 2017;376(22):2147–59.
14. von Minckwitz G, Huang C-S, Mano MS, Loibl S, Mamounas EP, Untch M, et al. Trastuzumab emtansine for residual invasive HER2-positive breast cancer. (KATHERINE). N Engl J Med. 2019;380:617–28.
15. Zarebczan Dull B, Neuman HB. Management of the axilla. Surg Clin North Am. 2013;93:429–44.
16. Rubio IT. Sentinel lymph node biopsy after neoadjuvant treatment in breast cancer: work in progress. Eur J Surg Oncol. 2016;42:326–32.
17. Krishnamurthy S, et al. Role of ultrasound-guided fine-needle aspiration of indeterminate and suspicious axillary lymph nodes in the initial staging of breast carcinoma. Cancer. 2002;95(5):982–8. https://doi.org/10.1002/cncr.10786.
18. Tahir M, et al. Preoperative axillary staging in breast cancer—saving time and resources. Breast J. 2008;4:369.
19. Alkuwari E, et al. Accuracy of fine-needle aspiration cytology of axillary lymph nodes in breast cancer patients. Cancer Cytopathol. 2008;114(2):89–93.
20. Mamounas EP, Brown A, Anderson S, et al. Sentinel node biopsy after neoadjuvant chemotherapy in breast cancer: results from National Surgical Adjuvant Breast and Bowel Project Protocol B-27. J Clin Oncol. 2005;23(12):2694–702.
21. Kelly, et al. Sentinel node identification and classification after neoadjuvant chemotherapy—systematic review and meta-analysis. Acad Radiol. 2009;16:551–63.
22. Geng C, et al. The feasibility and accuracy of sentinel lymph node biopsy in initially clinically node-negative breast cancer after neoadjuvant chemotherapy: a systematic review and meta-analysis. PLoS One. 2016;11(9):0162605.
23. Hunt KK, Yi M, et al. Sentinel lymph node surgery after neoadjuvant chemotherapy is accurate and reduces the need for axillary dissection in breast cancer patients. Ann Surg. 2009;250(4):558–66.
24. Boughey JC, Suman VJ, Mittendorf EA, et al. Sentinel lymph node surgery after neoadjuvant chemotherapy in patients with node-positive breast cancer: the ACOSOG Z1071 (Alliance) clinical trial. JAMA. 2013;310(14):1455–61.
25. Kuehn T, Bauerfeind I, Fehm T, Fleige B, Hausschild M, Helms G, et al. Sentinel-lymph-node biopsy in patients with breast cancer before and after neoadjuvant chemotherapy (SENTINA): a prospective, multicentre cohort study. Lancet Oncol. 2013;14:609–18.
26. Boileau JF, Poirier B, Basik M, Holloway CM, Gaboury L, Sideris L, et al. Sentinel node biopsy after neoadjuvant chemotherapy in biopsy-proven node-positive breast cancer: the SN FNAC study. J Clin Oncol. 2015;33:258–64.
27. Classe J-M, et al. Sentinel lymph node biopsy without axillary lymphadenectomy after neoadjuvant chemotherapy is accurate and safe for selected patients: the GANEA 2 study. Breast Cancer Res Treat. 2019;173(2):343–52.
28. El Hage Chehade H, et al. Is sentinel lymph node biopsy a viable alternative to complete axillary dissection following neoadjuvant chemotherapy in women with node-positive breast cancer at diagnosis? An updated meta-analysis involving 3,398 patients. Am J Surg. 2016;212(5):969–81.
29. Caudle AS, et al. Improved axillary evaluation following neoadjuvant therapy for patients with node-positive breast cancer using selective evaluation of clipped nodes: implementation of targeted axillary dissection. J Clin Oncol. 2016;34(10):1072–8.
30. Donker M, et al. Marking axillary lymph nodes with radioactive iodine seeds for axillary staging after neoadjuvant systemic treatment in breast cancer patients: the MARI procedure. Ann Surg. 2015;261(2):378–82.

31. van Nijnatten TJA, et al. A novel less-invasive approach for axillary staging after neoadjuvant chemotherapy in patients with axillary node-positive breast cancer by combining radioactive iodine seed localization in the Axilla with the sentinel node procedure (RISAS): a Dutch prospective multicenter validation study. Clin Breast Cancer. 2017;17:399–402..
32. Swarnkar PK, et al. The evolving role of marked lymph node biopsy (MLNB) and targeted axillary dissection (TAD) after neoadjuvant chemotherapy (NACT) for node-positive breast cancer: systematic review and pooled analysis. Cancers (Basel). 2021;13(7):1539.
33. Galimberti V, et al. Sentinel node biopsy after neoadjuvant treatment in breast cancer: five-year follow-up of patients with clinically node-negative or node-positive disease before treatment. Eur J Surg Oncol. 2016;42(3):361–8.
34. Nogi H, et al. Long-term follow-up of node-negative breast cancer patients evaluated via sentinel node biopsy after neoadjuvant chemotherapy. Clin Breast Cancer. 2017;17(8):644–9.
35. Kahler-Riberio-Fontana S, et al. Long-term standard sentinel node biopsy after neoadjuvant treatment in breast cancer: a single institution ten-year follow-up. Eur J Surg Oncol. 2021;47(4):804–12.
36. Martelli G, et al. Sentinel node biopsy alone or with axillary dissection in breast cancer patients after primary chemotherapy: long-term results of a Prospective Interventional Study. Ann Surg. 2020;276:e544.
37. Piltin MA, et al. Oncologic outcomes of sentinel lymph node surgery after neoadjuvant chemotherapy for node-positive breast cancer. Ann Surg Oncol. 2020;27(12):4795–801.
38. Wong SM, et al. Oncologic outcomes of sentinel lymph node surgery after neoadjuvant chemotherapy for node-positive breast cancer. Ann Surg Oncol. 2021;28(5):2621–9.
39. Moo T-A, et al. Is low-volume disease in the sentinel node after neoadjuvant chemotherapy an indication for axillary dissection? Ann Surg Onco. 2018;25(6):1488–94.

Addressing Node-Negative Axilla (N0) in Resource-Constrained Scenarios

11

Vani Parmar and Nita S. Nair

11.1 Introduction

Axillary lymph node dissection (ALND) for upfront operated node-negative axilla in breast cancer is now considered overtreatment due to the resultant morbidity and lifelong limitations to the affected limb. For operable early-stage breast cancer, sentinel lymph node biopsy (SLNB) is now the standard of care and pre-requisite to addressing the axilla completely.

11.2 Sentinel Lymph Node Biopsy

Sentinel lymph node biopsy consists of the dual-dye technique, with the use of any two non-interacting agents such as filtered radiocolloid-labelled Technetium 99 (^{99}Tc) or a coloured dye such as isosulphan blue, methylene blue, indocyanine green (ICG) dye, fluorescein dye or ferrous sulphate crystals (identified by magnetometer). The single-dye technique is associated with inferior identification rate compared with the dual-dye technique, although numerous centres have been showing good results with the use of ICG alone. The dye travels from the site of injection on the breast (intradermal/subdermal over the tumour or sub-areolar or intra-parenchymal, peri-tumoural) via the lymphatic system to the axillary lymph nodes (LNs). Evidence suggests that the dye injected in any site in the breast, as in intradermal, subdermal over tumour or sub-areolar or intra parenchymal, or peri-tumoural, all successfully identify the sentinel lymph node (SLN) [1].

V. Parmar (✉) · N. S. Nair
Breast Surgical Oncology, Tata Memorial Centre and Homi Bhabha National Institute, Mumbai, India

Chintamani (ed.), *Sentinel Node Biopsy in Breast Cancer*,
https://doi.org/10.1007/978-81-322-3994-9_11

The principle behind SLNB is based on systematic drainage of tumor cells via the lymphatic pathways to the first echelon axillary node with adjacent palpably enlarged nodes in level I of axilla, all together called the 'sentinel node(s)', with adjacent palpably enlarged nodes also being considered part of this first level draining LN, followed by sequential drainage into the level II and III LNs. The main difference in the various techniques of SLNB is based on the size of particles and the method of detecting the node that has picked up the specific agent and has its own specific advantages and limitations. The radiocolloid-labelled ^{99}Tc requires a hand-held gamma probe for identifying the SLN and access to a nuclear medicine department wherein the radioactive source is prepared fresh on the day of surgery. The filtering and tagging of the ^{99}Tc happen before injecting as it has a definite half-life and hence needs to be injected 2 h before surgery. In certain cases, the injection can be given on the previous day but at a much higher dose and larger molecular size so the travel through the lymphatics is slower. The hand-held gamma probe used to identify the node with radioactivity is an expensive investment but is useful nonetheless. The cost may be a limitation in certain centres treating breast cancer. Also, more importantly, the radioactive source itself is not available in many areas and thus may limit the use of radiocolloid. There are, as of today, 359 nuclear medicine centres in India [2]. Breast cancer surgery still continues to remain in the domain of general surgeons in most cities, although relatively, the specialist breast cancer centres have increased significantly in the last decade or so, much more than the increase in nuclear medicine facilities. These facilities are therefore largely unable to cater to the various medical colleges, cancer centres and small-sized hospitals, nursing homes and private centres that are treating breast cancer in India.

A combination of blue dye and radiocolloid, approximately 18.5–30 Mbq (0.5–0.8 mCi) of radiopharmaceutical, injected at the primary site, was also described by Glass and Morton [3] for dynamic imaging to differentiate SNLs and non-SNLs. Since then, radiocolloid injection has remained the mainstay of SLNB and has been one agent that has stood the test of time; it has been paired with various other coloured agents for visual localisation of the SN.

Targeted SLNB can be performed using various coloured dyes. Patent blue or isosulphan blue is probably the first reported agent to be used as early as in 1990 [4, 5]. These were validation procedures with complete nodal basin clearance after SLNB in all cases and reported identification in 82% of cases with 1% false-negative rate (FNR). Subsequently, the technique was used in many other cancers including breast cancer [6], colon cancer, lung cancer and virtually all solid neoplasms that have lymphatic spread. Isosulphan blue dye or patent blue is a vital dye with rapid clearance through the kidney. It is an inert agent, but can sometimes cause anaphylactic reactions. It is available as an anhydrous powder that has to be dissolved in distilled water to prepare a 1% strength dye and requires solution to be prepared and bottled in ampoules followed by sterilisation in small portions to allow easy use pre-operatively. The main limitations of its use in India are limited availability and higher cost. It can result in post-operative 'blue urine' that patients should be informed about pre-operatively.

At a much lower cost, a popular alternative to isosulphan blue is methylene blue which is easily available over the counter and can be accessed even in the remotest parts of the country at a very nominal cost. The sterilised dye can be used instead of vital blue to perform SLNB and has been tested now in many studies and found to be equally effective in identifying blue lymphatics and blue stained SLNs. It also has property of renal excretion, but can cause significant skin necrosis when used intradermally. Hence, it mandates for excision of the area of the skin at site of intradermal methylene blue infiltration.

Most studies of SLNB have shown that even though a SLN is hypothetically a single node, more than one SN are identified in majority of cases, sometimes even up to eight LNs. In fact, it has been observed that the higher the number of SNs identified, the lower is the reported FNR, with a suggestion that more than three SNs are required to reduce FNR to an acceptable level [7]. Additionally these SNs are mostly situated in the lower realms of the axilla. An FNR, as reported in a large prospective randomised trial [8], is as much as 9.8% for a median pT size of 1.2 cm and 28% nodal disease, with no detriment in overall survival if axillary clearance was omitted with a negative SLN [9]. These studies established that an FNR below 10% is considered acceptable for early-stage breast cancer. Also since 2.3% of the SLN were identified as palpable LNs with no dye uptake, the SLN subsequently included radioactive, coloured and large palpable LNs.

11.3 Axillary Sampling

Axillary sampling is a method of identifying a group of LNs in the lower axilla and can be done by palpation, anatomical dissection or blue dye-guided excision; it may or may not include the surrounding axillary fat as the specific LNs are removed.

The principle of axillary sampling is based on the premise that:

(a) SLNs are mainly detected in the lower realms of the lower axilla.
(b) The higher the number of SLNs removed, the lower the false-negative rate.
(c) Swedish 5-node sampling had a low FNR and supported its feasibility.
(d) Four-node axillary sampling (4NAS) was already accepted as standard in Nottingham Breast Unit.
(e) Identifying and excising fat with LNs in the lower axilla would negate subjectivity of nodal pickup by palpation alone, improve the learning curve and would have least possibility of missing an involved node in the lower axilla or axillary tail.
(f) Most axillary reverse-mapping LNs are found above the first intercostobrachial nerve, and sampling nodes are situated below the intercostobrachial nerve, thereby effectively sparing the lymphatic drainage of arm [10].
(g) Would not require targeting the SN by any of the above techniques if proven equivalent and reliable.

With this background and premise, a prospective comparative study of low axillary sampling (LAS) and SLNB was carried out on 478 Indian women with clinically node-negative early-stage breast cancer at a large tertiary referral centre. The results showed equal efficacy of LAS and SLNB in predicting axillary nodal status, with FNRs of 10.5% (95% CI, 6.6–16.2) for LAS and 12.7% (95% CI, 8.1–19.4) for SLNB ($p = 0.56$), comparable to the FNR of SLNB reported in the NSABP B32 study (9.8%, 95% CI 7.8–12.2). When palpable nodes in the vicinity were excluded from the SLNB criteria, limiting it to targeted node alone, the FNR was high at 29.0% (95% CI, 22.5–36.6), indicating that much of the accuracy of SLNB is derived from the inclusion of the surrounding palpable nodes [11].

This technique of LAS, which is an anatomically guided excision, has since then been accepted as the standard and practiced routinely in early-stage breast cancer at Tata Memorial Centre. We subsequently audited the data in 623 women, with cN0 and cN1 soft node, and operable breast cancer, treated during 2012–2018. All 623 underwent LAS (no blue dye) followed by FS, and those positive on FS had completion ALND. If final HPR of LAS was later positive, ALND was completed later. Overall 304 patients (48.7%) had positive LAS LN on FS that were correctly identified and a subsequent ALND was done. Median LN dissected in LAS on FS was 5 [1–9], and 21 positive axillae were effectively missed (FNR 21/325 = 6.5%) [12].

With the validation of LAS in early-stage breast cancer, the technique was further extended and tested in post-neo-adjuvant chemotherapy clinically N0 (cN0) axilla in locally advanced breast cancer. In both upfront and post-chemotherapy situation, no pre-operative or pre-chemotherapy ultrasound of the axilla was done. As practiced in many centres across India, no axillary nodal FNAC or core biopsy was practiced, and the axillary node was not clipped. The axillae deemed clinically node-negative after chemotherapy were subjected to LAS [13].

The study showed that post-NACT, SLNB (targeted node with palpable suspicious adjacent node) has an FNR of 19.7% (95% CI one-sided upper limit 24). Using the LAS technique of removing lower axillary nodes and fat defined by anatomical boundaries improves FNR to 9.9% with a one-sided 95% CI upper limit 12.8 ($p < 0.001$) with 94.0% negative predictive value (NPV) and can be considered as a suitable alternative in countries with limited resources. The yield of LNs was higher in the study with a median of 7 LNs in LAS and 5 LNs in targeted SN with palpable nodes. Limiting the technique to only targeted SN retrieval resulted in median 2 SNs identified with an FNR of 31.6%, and NPV of 84.1%, indicating an unacceptable high risk of leaving behind disease in the axilla if it were to be followed for deciding axillary clearance post-chemotherapy. Currently, a limited axillary surgery in a post-NACT node-negative axilla is still not a standard of care, although the results of LAS study suggests safety of moving to LAS in post-chemotherapy N0 axilla to decide the fate of the rest of the axillary nodes.

The ALLIANCE Z10071 trial enrolled 756 women with clinical T0–4, N1–2, M0 breast cancer and had received neo-adjuvant chemotherapy. Of these 756 women, 663 were cN1 initially, of which 84% became node negative post chemotherapy (ycN0). The dual technique had superior results, and examining at least three SLNs was recommended to reduce FNR significantly from 21.1% with two SNs to 9.1% with three LNs. A finding very similar to that of the LAS technique, with examination of at least three LNs, reduced the FNR to 8.8%, raising the possibility of the LAS technique being accepted as a feasible and attractive alternative to SLNB in these subsets of patients for LMIC [14]. Studies are now also ongoing considering RT instead of surgery for the rest of the axillary nodes in this subset of individuals with a higher risk of breast cancer after chemotherapy (ALLIANCE A011202), the results of which are still awaited.

11.4 Omitting ALND in pN1–2 SLNs

Five landmark trials evaluated the role of axillary conservation in women with SLN-positive axilla. Three studies, ACOSOG Z0011 [15], IBCSG 23–01 [16] and ATTRM-048-13-200 [17], compared ALND with sentinel lymph node dissection (SLND) to SLND alone, and two studies, namely, OTOASOR [18] and AMAROS [19], compared ALND with axillary radiotherapy (aRT). A systematic review by Schmidt-Hansen et al. [20] reported no detriment on recurrence or survival. However, the quality of data is deemed as weak, and there was considerable variation in the population included across the studies; thus, they suggested that a combination of the results from these is not adequate to avoid an ALND in all subgroups. High-risk populations were grossly under-represented in the landmark studies evaluating omission of ALND in women with 1–2 SLN-positive EBC. Also, previous studies have suggested that 15–30% of clinically node-negative patients will develop axillary failure if the axilla is left untreated by either radiotherapy or dissection. Despite this, many Indian centres were keen on applying the same to our population of patients with early-stage breast cancer and to change practices by avoiding completion axillary clearance even if 1–2 SLNs were positive.

In lieu of the continuing debate, centres have audited the outcome data of women with 1–2 positive LNs (LN+) in India and compared the outcome of patients in the ACOZOG Z0011 trial. One such retrospective audit was a comparison published from Tata Memorial Centre, Mumbai [12], wherein all cN0 early-stage breast cancer patients, who were operated from 2013 to 2018 and underwent LAS, were evaluated. Of the 2350 cN0 patients, 687 (29%) had LN+ on final histopathology, of whom 597 (86.9%) had 1–2 LN+, 40 (5.8%) patients had 3 LN+, and 50 (7.3%) had four or more positive nodes. The TMC audit [12] also evaluated the percentage of additional LN+ in the ALND group and compared it to the ACOSOG Z11 trial population. Of the 2350 cN0 patients with EBC who underwent LAS, 687 (29%) had LN+ on final histopathology. Overall 656 women underwent ALND, and additional disease in the rest of the axilla was noted in 190/597 (31.82%) in those with 1–2 LN+, in 18/40 (45%) with three nodes positive on LAS and in 37/50 (74%) in those with four or more nodes in LAS. The odds for having axilla positivity for patients with three LNs were 1.8 times higher than those for patients with 1–2 LNs. Patients with ≥4 LN were 6.6 times significantly more likely to have axilla positivity than patients with 1–2 LNs. There was a 48% increase in probability of additional disease in the rest of the axilla with every additional LN+ in LAS.

This study showed that demographic features in the ACOSOG Z11 were starkly different from those seen in Indian patients. The ACOSOG Z11 patient cohort was different with a median pT of 1.7 cm, 30% grade III tumours and 45% with micrometastasis in LNs, as compared to the Indian patient cohort with 3 cm median pT size, 73.7% grade 3 tumours and 99.2% with macro-metastatic LNs in the ACOSOG cohort, versus 3 cm median pT size tumours, 99.2% with macro-metastatic LNs, and 73.7% grade 3 tumours in the Indian cohort, respectively. In the Indian cohort, 31.8% of the 1–2 LN+ had additional LN+ on ALND. Keeping in mind the difference in clinicopathological features between the Indian cohorts and ACOZOG Z0011, with a third of women having additional LN+ on ALND, it may not be appropriate to apply the results and inference of the ACOSOG Z0011 trial directly to the Indian population and to address the rest of the axilla with surgery. Possibly, only a select subset of patients who match the trial population of the ACOSOG Z11 could be offered observation of the axilla, and validated nomograms can be used to identify high-risk patients. Similarly, Agarwal et al. [21] also recommend an ALND if SLNB/LAS is positive, citing reasons of higher-grade tumour, younger age, more hormone-negative cancers and macro-metastatic disease with extra-nodal invasion in such patients.

11.5 Factors That Predict the Risk of Non-SLN Positive

Van la Parra et al. [22] and Toshikawa et al. [23] evaluated the risk of NSLN and concluded that we must thus be able to predict which group is at risk of NSLN metastasis in the case of 1–2 SNs positive when making decisions regarding omitting ALND. Multiple studies have evaluated risk factors for NSLN metastasis, including T size, grade, number of positive SLN, macro-metastases, lymphovascular invasion and extra-nodal involvement [24]. The most consistent have been LVI and ENI. Tumours with positive LVI have 1.5 times increased risk, whereas those with positive ENI have 3.6 times increased risk of having NSLN metastasis [12]. Various nomograms addressing the role risk on NSLN metastasis in women with 1–2 SLNs are available but need to be validated for the Indian cohort before being recommended for use [25].

Conflict of Interest Statement None of the authors have any conflict of interest to be declared.

References

1. Celliers L, Mann GB. Alternative sites of injection for sentinel lymph node biopsy in breast cancer. ANZ J Surg. 2003;73(8):600–4.
2. https://www.aerb.gov.in/images/PDF/NuclearMedicine/RSD1.pdf.
3. Glass EC, Essner R, Morton DL. Kinetics of three lymphoscintigraphic agents in patients with cutaneous melanoma. J Nucl Med. 1998;39:1185–90.
4. Morton D, Cagle L, Wong J, et al. Intraoperative lymphatic mapping and selective lymphadenectomy: technical details of a new procedure for clinical stage I melanoma. In: Presented at the annual meeting of the Society of Surgical Oncology, Washington, DC; 1990.
5. Morton DL, Wen DR, Wong JH, et al. Technical details of intraoperative lymphatic mapping for early stage melanoma. Arch Surg. 1992;392-99:392.
6. Giuliano AE, Kirgan DM, Guenther JM, et al. Lymphatic mapping and sentinel lymphadenectomy for breast cancer. Ann Surg. 1994;220:391–8.
7. Chagpar AB, Scoggins CR, Martin RCG II, Carlson DJ, Laidley AL, El-Eid SE, McGlothin TQ, McMasters KM, for the University of Louisville Breast Sentinel Lymph Node Study Investigators. Are 3 sentinel nodes sufficient? Arch Surg. 2007;142:456–60.

8. Krag DN, Anderson SJ, Julian TB, et al; National Surgical Adjuvant Breast and Bowel Project. Technical outcomes of sentinel-lymph-node resection and conventional axillary-lymph-node dissection in patients with clinically node-negative breast cancer: results from the NSABP B-32 randomised phase III trial. Lancet Oncol 2007;8(10):881–8.
9. Krag DN, Anderson SJ, Julian TB, et al. Sentinel-lymph-node resection compared with conventional axillary-lymph-node dissection in clinically node-negative patients with breast cancer: overall survival findings from the NSABP B-32 randomised phase 3 trial. Lancet Oncol. 2010;11(10):927–33.
10. Ahmed M, Rubio IT, Kovacs T, Klimberg VS, Douek M. Systematic review of axillary reverse mapping in breast cancer. Br J Surg. 2016;103(3):170–8.
11. Parmar V, Hawaldar R, Nair NS, et al. Sentinel node biopsy versus low axillary sampling in women with clinically node negative operable breast cancer. Breast. 2013;22(6):1081–6. https://doi.org/10.1016/j.breast.2013.06.006. pii: S0960-9776(13)00171-9. PubMed PMID: 23948301.
12. Reddy A, Nair NS, Mokal S, et al. Can we avoid axillary lymph node dissection (ALND) in patients with 1–2 positive sentinel/low axillary lymph nodes (SLN/LAS+) in the Indian setting? Indian J SurgOncol. 2021;12:272. https://doi.org/10.1007/s13193-021-01297-6.
13. Parmar V, Nair NS, Vanmali V, et al. Sentinel node biopsy versus low axillary sampling in predicting nodal status of postchemotherapy axilla in women with breast cancer. JCO Glob Oncol. 2020;6:1546–53.
14. Boughey JC, Suman VJ, Mittendorf EA, et al. Sentinel lymph node surgery after neoadjuvant chemotherapy in patients with node-positive breast cancer: the ACOSOG Z1071 (Alliance) clinical trial. JAMA. 2013;310:1455–61.
15. Giuliano AE, Hunt KK, Ballman KV, et al. Axillary dissection vs no axillary dissection in women with invasive breast cancer and sentinel node metastasis: a randomized clinical trial. JAMA. 2011;305(6):569–75.
16. Galimberti V, Cole BF, Zurrida S, et al. International Breast Cancer Study Group. Axillary dissection versus no axillary dissection in patients with sentinel-node micrometastases (IBCSG 23-01): a phase 3 randomised controlled trial. Lancet Oncol. 2013;14(4):297–305.
17. Sola MS, Alberro JA, Fraile M, et al. Complete axillary lymph node dissection versus clinical follow-up in breast cancer patients with sentinel node micrometastasis: final results from the multicenter clinical trial AATRM 048/13/2000. Ann Surg Oncol. 2013;20:120–7.
18. Savolt A, Musonda P, Matrai Z, et al. Optimal treatment of the axilla after positive sentinel lymph node biopsy in early invasive breast cancer. Early results of the OTOASOR trial. Orv Hetil. 2013;154:1934–42.
19. Straver ME, Meijnen P, van Tienhoven G, et al. Sentinel node identification rate and nodal involvement in the EORTC 10981-22023 AMAROS trial. Ann Surg Oncol. 2010;17:1854–61.
20. Schmidt-Hansen M, et al. Axillary surgery in women with sentinel node-positive operable breast cancer: a systematic review with meta-analyses. Springerplus. 2016;5(1):85.
21. Agarwal G, Gambhir S, Lal P, Krishnani N, Rajan S. Avoidance of axillary dissection in cN0 breast cancer patients with metastatic sentinel lymph node(s) using ACOSOG Z-0011 criteria: is it appropriate for Indian patients? J Clin Oncol. 2015;33(28 Suppl):62.
22. Van la Parra RF, Peer PG, Ernst MF, et al. Meta-analysis of predictive factors for non-sentinel lymph node metastases in breast cancer patients with a positive SLN. Eur J Surg Oncol. 2011;37:290–9.
23. Toshikawa C, Koyama Y, Nagahashi M, et al. Predictive factors for non-sentinel lymph node metastasis in the case of positive sentinel lymph node metastasis in two or fewer nodes in breast cancer. J Clin Med Res. 2015;7:620–6.
24. Gooch J, King TA, Eaton A. The extent of extracapsular extension may influence the need for axillary lymph node dissection in patients with T1-T2 breast cancer. Ann Surg Oncol. 2014;21:2897–903.
25. Reddy A, Nair NS, Mokal S, et al. Validation of nomograms to predict non-sentinel lymph node metastasis after positive sentinel lymph node in breast cancer: Indian cohort background. J Clin Oncol. 2020;38(15_Suppl):568.

MIX
Papier aus verantwortungsvollen Quellen
Paper from responsible sources
FSC® C105338

If you have any concerns about our products,
you can contact us on
ProductSafety@springernature.com

In case Publisher is established outside the EU,
the EU authorized representative is:
Springer Nature Customer Service Center GmbH
Europaplatz 3, 69115 Heidelberg, Germany

Printed by Libri Plureos GmbH
in Hamburg, Germany